The Crying Book

The Crying Book

✦ ✦ ✦

HEATHER CHRISTLE

Catapult 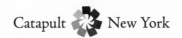 New York

The Crying Book

The author has tried to re-create events, locales, and conversations based on her own memories and those of others. In some instances, in order to maintain their anonymity, certain names, characteristics, and locations have been changed.

ISBN: 978-1-948226-44-8

Cover design by Nicole Caputo
Book design by Jordan Koluch

This artist was awarded the Ohio Arts Council's Individual Excellence Award for 2018.

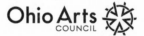

Catapult titles are distributed to the trade by Publishers Group West
Phone: 866-400-5351

Library of Congress Control Number: 2019935113

Printed in the United States of America
3 5 7 9 10 8 6 4 2

Author's Note

This book began five years ago with an idle idea about what it might look like to make a map of every place I'd ever cried, an idea I carried into conversation with friends, not knowing how many years and pages would grow around it, not knowing how that growth would change the way I view tears.

These pages are a record of that time, of what I learned. And go on learning.

Throughout this work, when I have talked with my friends about crying, I have felt the gifts of their intelligence, compassion, humor, and patience. It would have been, I think, impossible to write this book without their company. Their names appear in these pages informally, as they do in my mind and our conversations.

Of the many circumstances in my life for which I feel gratitude, these friendships shine with a particular brightness. They make me look eagerly to the future, to imagine all the conversations to come.

◆ ◆ ◆

I suppose some people can weep softly and become more beautiful, but after a real cry, most people are hideous, as if they've grown a spare and diseased face beneath the one you know, leaving very little room for the eyes. Or they look as if they've been beaten. We look. I look. Once, in fifth grade, I cried at school for a reason I cannot recall, and afterward a popular boy—rattail, skateboard—told me I looked *like a druggie*, and I was so pleased to be seen I made him repeat it.

◆ ◆ ◆

Ovid would prefer that I and other women restrain ourselves:

There is no limit to art: in weeping, you need to
    be comely,
Learn how to turn on the tears still keeping
    proper control.[1]

◆ ◆ ◆

The length of the cry matters. I especially value an extended session, which gives me time to become curious, to look in the mirror, to observe my physical sadness. A truly powerful cry can withstand even this scientific activity. You lurch toward the bathroom, head hunched over, tucked in, and then gather your nerve to lift your gaze toward the mirror, where you see your hiccoughing breath shake your shoulders, your nose like a lifelong drunk's. It may interest you for a while to touch your swollen face, to peer into one bloodshot eye and another, but the beauty's really in the movement, in watching your mouth try to swallow despair. It is not easy, after looking, to convince the crying you mean it no harm, but with quiet and with patience—you are Jane Goodall with the chimpanzees—the crying will slowly get used to you. It will return.

◆ ◆ ◆

To cry or not to cry is sometimes a choice, and no telling which is the better. Not true—if you are alone, or with only one other, cry. To cry with more people present, concludes the International Study of Adult Crying, can lead to a worsening mood, though that may depend on others' reactions. You can be made to feel ashamed. Most frequently criers report others responding with compassion, or what the study categorizes as "comfort words, comfort arms, and understanding."[2] If you are alone, comfort arms are still available; you hold yourself together.

+ + +

It is fortunate to have a nose. Hard to feel you are too tragic a figure when the tears mix with snot. There is no glamour in honking.

+ + +

Once I was unexpectedly dumped in public. A campus parking lot one afternoon. I put all my crying into my mouth, felt it shake while I stalked to the car, inside which I let the crying move north to my eyes and south to my heaving gut. The car is a private crying area. If you see a person crying *near* a car, you may need to offer help. If you see a person crying *inside* a car, you know they are already held.

+ + +

Twice I cried hysterically while driving. Once, sixteen, and without money for the toll or a sense of how I might live the next day. Once, twenty-one, and mid-move, with a car full of belongings and the sudden apprehension that I had driven an hour in the wrong direction. If you cry in the car while it's raining, it feels like the windshield wipers should tend too to your face. Comfort words, comfort arms, comfort swipe.

✦ ✦ ✦

I cried when I heard Alice Oswald recite *Memorial*, her excavation of the *Iliad*, marking each warrior's death. I cried while a friend held her new son and told me about a conversation she'd had with her own mother, Sheila. My friend had realized that one day she'd no longer need to wash her boy's feet, and the thought wounded her. "Mom," she asked Sheila, "do you still miss that?" Sheila replied, "I'd give anything to wash my son's feet." As I write this down it sounds utterly servile. At the time I could not help but weep. Motherhood gets me. I cry whenever I watch a representation—whether fictional or no—of birth. I have also cried at the gym, on the elliptical, watching a trailer for some dumb and heartbreaking movie. I waited until my sister's car was one hundred yards into her move to Maine, and then I cried. I cried in front of a crowd—mortifying—while reading a poem I wrote for my dead friend Bill. He would have laughed. He would have liked it.

✦ ✦ ✦

Do you remember the hopelessness of watching a parent cry?

❖ ❖ ❖

When Bill died I went to a museum and cried.

❖ ❖ ❖

I do not allow roadkill to make me cry anymore.

❖ ❖ ❖

When I was young my nose used to bleed so badly at times that when it finally began to clot, my nasal passages would clog up, and I'd cry tears of blood.

❖ ❖ ❖

There are chemical differences between emotional tears and those produced by physical irritation. People who sniff emotional tears show decreased sexual arousal.[3] Once I started to cry during sex, not about the sex, but rather the mawkish Belle and Sebastian song playing on the stereo. People cry in response to art, most frequently to music. Poetry gets claimed second.[4] People can even cry about architecture.[5]

❖ ❖ ❖

The first thing you ever did was cry. According to William Derham, writing in the Royal Society's *Philosophical*

Transactions in 1708, at least one human began crying while still in the womb, which led to skeptical responses from correspondents who thought the noise must have been a "Groaking of the Guts, or Womb, or the Effect of . . . Feminine Imagination."[6] "Scarce a Day," insisted Derham, "in all the five Weeks escaped without Crying little or much," though the boy was, he went on to say, "since its Birth, a very quiet Child."[7]

+ + +

I met Bill at a poetry reading when we were both still living in New York City, and we made plans to meet up, talk poems, try a friendship. Eventually we rendezvoused at a lousy bar near Union Square. "I'm pregnant," I told him, and ordered a drink.

+ + +

After the abortion I bled for weeks. One evening so much it frightened me. I called the clinic and they said to go to the emergency room, but I didn't have any money. I called Bill and he said he'd come over. He spent the night in my bed while I cried and bled and cried. It was the only time we kissed.

+ + +

I speak to Lisa and Lisa speaks of parallel crying, the crying that comes alongside art but not precisely from it. Plot does not jerk the tears from you; some other force corresponds. This pleases me, as I have always preferred parallel lines to perpendicular ones. Perpendicular lines are Chekhovian; the introduced gun goes off. Parallel lines are Hitchcockian; the present bomb is enough.

◆ ◆ ◆

Most crying happens at night. People cry out of fatigue. But how horrible it is to hear someone say, "She's just tired!" Tired, yes, certainly, but *just?* There is nothing just about it.

◆ ◆ ◆

I remember watching my mother cry one brief winter day, though I can't recall why she was so sad. Perhaps there was no reason, only an atmosphere: my merchant mariner father's absence at sea, the endless demanding presence of my sister and myself. I remember the brightness of the room, sunlight assailing every surface.

◆ ◆ ◆

In the immediate aftermath of the massacre at Kent State in 1970, one witness mistook the tears of students crying at the deaths of their classmates for tears produced by gas—the *lacrymator* the National Guard had weaponized against protestors. Years later, she told an interviewer:

I still was convinced, for some crazy reason, that there was just tear gas. [...] I had no clue where the ambulances were going or why there were so many of them and why they were so loud and moving so fast and why people were crying so hard and hugging each other and being so hysterical. So I kept walking. [...] And they drove me home. Shelly and Mark drove me home. And my mother was standing in the driveway crying, waiting for me, thinking that I was one of the dead people at Kent. And she was crying. [...] I don't even remember what happened after I got into my parents' house, other than there was a lot of crying on my mother's part. And I don't remember crying at all.[8]

+ + +

The National Guard threw tear gas canisters at the students—"laid some gas," to use their phrase—and the students threw them back, an act of protection and defiance: *No, thank you; we don't want this.* Retaliating, escalating, the soldiers aimed their M1 rifles.

+ + +

Among the remedies for tear gas—a cold-water rinse, a turn to face the wind—the command to *remain calm* sounds hardest to put into practice.

In the photo that came to represent the massacre, a fourteen-year-old girl kneels beside the body of a slain student, her whole body an anguished question.

+ + +

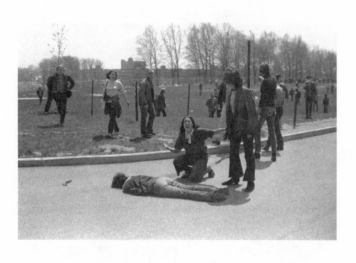

+ + +

Tears are a sign of powerlessness, a "woman's weapon." It has been a very long war.

+ + +

Yi-Fei Chen, a design student in the Netherlands, literalized the metaphor after a demanding professor made her cry. She constructed a brass gun that collects, freezes, and shoots tears: tiny icy bullets. Chen presented the object at her graduation, where she accepted an invitation to take aim at the head of her department.[9]

◆ ◆ ◆

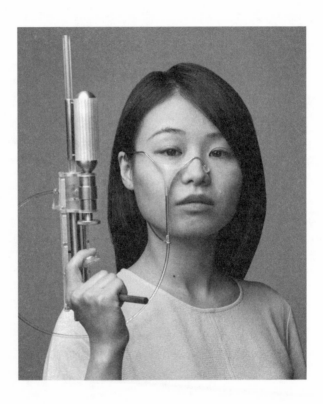

◆ ◆ ◆

I get irritable reading the "crying expert" Ad Vingerhoets's deeply researched and meticulous book *Why Only Humans*

Weep, for what feels like his aggressive lack of compassion or wonder, but then am intrigued by a sudden pronouncement: "All tears are real tears," he says, though some may be "insincere."[10]

We scrutinize the tears of other people for their sincerity. We can even doubt the sincerity of our own. In *Letters to Wendy's,* Joe Wenderoth writes of a child's strategic crying at the fast food restaurant:

> His mother explained to me that this was no true grief—this was pretend grief. This was grief, she said, designed to get something. And I thought, have I anything but pretend grief? And I asked myself what I meant, in these daily excretions of pretend grief, to acquire? And I couldn't answer. And I felt true grief.[11]

Here is another term for pretend grief: *cry-hustling,* coined by the poet Chelsey Minnis (a *nom,* by the way, *de plume,* or perhaps *de guerre*).

> A woman is cry-hustling a man & it is very fun.
> You have to cry-hustle because it is good to
>   cry-hustle ...
> And there's nothing else you can do.

11

THE CRYING BOOK

Because no one will agree to any of your reason-
      able statements ...
And they have to counter-argue ...
Then you just have to break down and cry-
      hustle ...[12]

+ + +

The tears of white women are subject to specific scrutiny, because their weaponization has so often meant violence toward people of color, and black people in particular. The tears could be real, by which I mean *physically present*, or imagined, *metaphorical*. Whether they exist on the face or in the mind, the tears of a white woman can shift a room's gravity. They set others falling to help her, to correct and punish those who would dare make her weep.

+ + +

As far as words go, *crying* is louder and *weeping* is wetter. When people explain the difference between the two to English-language learners they say that weeping is more formal, can sound archaic in everyday speech. You can hear this in their past tenses—the plainness of *cried*, the velvet cloak of *wept*. I remember arguing once with a teacher who insisted *dreamt* was incorrect, *dreamed* the only proper option. She was wrong, of course, in both philological and moral ways, and ever since I've felt a peculiar attachment to the *t*'s of the past: *weep, wept, sleep, slept, leave, left.* There's a finality there, a quiet completion, of which *d* has never dreamt.

❖   ❖   ❖

In his poem "Weeping," Ross Gay traces the etymology of the word from the proto-Indo-European root *wab-* through an imagined progression, pretending it

> means the precise sound of a flower bud
>
> unwrapping, and the tiny racket a seed makes
> cracking open in the dark . . .[13]

❖   ❖   ❖

Some mornings I awake with an enormous sensation inside me and cannot identify whether the urge is to cry or write a poem or fuck someone. All at once? My body has cross-indexed the impulse.

❖   ❖   ❖

I have not cried for some days when one morning I wake much earlier than usual. We have just moved into a new house and—because I am not yet accustomed to the skylight above the bed—the sound of rain against it stands between me and a return to sleep. In the kitchen, while I wait for coffee to brew, the BBC World Service tells the story of a man, L.D., whose ship capsized during World War II. Their distress signals mistakenly ignored, the surviving sailors floated for days in their life vests. When the sharks arrived they fed first on the dead, then the living. L.D. says there was nothing you could do beyond hoping you weren't next.

It's still so dark out that there's no real point in pulling back the curtains, but I do anyway, making the lit room visible to anyone else awake at this hour, and at the same time locating within myself the knowledge that I could not have reached such acceptance. Knowing that I would have given up.

After days of dehydration, one sailor slipped out of his life vest and swam down into the Pacific, believing in his delirium that the ship's water supply was within reach. He surfaced, ecstatic with having satisfied his thirst, and soon died, the brown foam at his mouth a mark of the salt water he'd swallowed.

At last, after four days of misery, a navy plane spotted the men. I wonder whether when the rescue crew at last pulled him to safety, L.D. wanted to cry with joy, whether his body would have had any water left for tears.[14]

+ + +

One night in the nursery, a boy sits crying. He has found his shadow and is desperately trying to re-adhere it to his body with soap, but cannot get it to stick back on again. When the sleeping girl wakes, a series of questions leads her to realize the boy is motherless. This shocks her into utter sympathy.

> WENDY. Peter!
> (*She leaps out of bed to put her arms round him, but he draws back; he does not know why, but he knows he must draw back.*)
> PETER. You mustn't touch me.
> WENDY. Why?
> PETER. No one must ever touch me.
> WENDY. Why?
> PETER. I don't know.
> (*He is never touched by any one in the play.*)
> WENDY. No wonder you were crying.
> PETER. I wasn't crying. But I can't get my shadow to stick on.[15]

+ + +

The denial of crying by a tear-streaked person is such a commonplace that it has become a joke. Look up "I'm not crying" on YouTube and the first few hundred results display people—very often children at a school talent show—singing the comic song by Flight of the Conchords, in which they blame their tears on the rain. I am growing to hate this song. It is in the way of my finding evidence of people actually crying, actually denying it. However hard I look all I find is this unfunny music.

✦ ✦ ✦

When I was five, I auditioned to play Wendy in *Peter Pan*, a part the children's summer theater company predictably assigned to an older girl. The announcement brought me very close to tears. Then they declared that the part of Tinker Bell would be played by my younger sister. I was to be "a fairy." I was to be a very sad, very wet fairy.

✦ ✦ ✦

The following year, in *Alice in Wonderland*, they cast me as the understudy to the small Alice: not the large Alice who weeps gallons of tears, but the shrunken one who nearly drowns in them. I spent the whole summer praying for calamity to befall the real small Alice, but she came to no harm. Instead, I performed in my other role: a centipede dancing insignificantly in the flower garden.

✦ ✦ ✦

In those years I was entranced by *The Wizard of Oz*, the first movie I ever saw on VHS, and loved to act the story out with my family. I remember insisting, during one game, that my mother—the Wicked Witch of the West—had to stay in the kitchen (her castle), while I skipped down the Yellow Brick Road to my Emerald City bedroom. My dolls were Munchkins, my sister the Scarecrow. I don't remember whether my father was there. He might have been the Tin Man; he might have been at sea.

◆ ◆ ◆

I fear that to write so much about crying will tempt a universal law of irony to invite tragedy into my life.

◆ ◆ ◆

A folk tale "common to ... country people belonging to the States of New York and Ohio," and recounted in an 1898 issue of *The Journal of American Folklore* mocks those who would cry at the thought of some possible future sorrow:

> Once there was a girl. One day her mother came into the kitchen and found the girl sitting crying with all her heart. The mother said, "Why, what is the matter?" The girl replied, "Oh, I was thinking. And I thought how someday perhaps I might be married and how I might have a baby, and then I thought how one day when it would be asleep

in its cradle the oven lid would fall on it and kill it," and she began to cry again.[16]

◆ ◆ ◆

Some people think of reading poems and stories as a way to practice responding to imagined circumstances, without having to risk the dangers of real life.

◆ ◆ ◆

Some people will write about one thing as a way of not writing about something else. Like Tony Tost:

> I don't know how to talk about my biological father, so I am going to describe the lake: it's blue, with swans.[17]

◆ ◆ ◆

It does not have to be swans. It could be elephants, as it is for Amy Lawless:

> When an elephant dies
> Sometimes all you have to do is be there
> And no one will judge you
> If you don't say something witty.

Sometimes when an elephant dies
I want to grab a bunch of scientists
And one scientist will wipe the tear
Out of the elephant's eye
And say "I can explain" and draw the bone
From the mouth of the living.[18]

✦ ✦ ✦

People have long made occasional reports of elephants weeping emotional tears, though for just as long skeptical observers have retorted that the animals cry only in response to physical pain. Whether or not it actually cries, the elephant is famous for its mourning. In 1999, Damimi, a seventy-two-year-old captive elephant, "died of grief," following the death of her younger elephant friend, who died while giving birth. According to the BBC, "Zoo officials said she shed tears over her friend's body, then stood still in her enclosure for days."[19] Eventually she starved.

✦ ✦ ✦

Such behavior is not limited to elephants in captivity. In the wild, writes one ecologist, "Mothers often are observed grieving over their dead child for days after the death, alternately trying to bring the baby back to life and caressing and touching the corpse."[20] The word I have seen people use most frequently to describe the way elephants examine the bones of another when a herd comes across a skeleton is *reverent.*

✦ ✦ ✦

It is hard to say, sometimes, whether tears are the product of physical or emotional pain. Take, for instance, this account of a white man hunting an elephant in South Africa in the late 1800s. At this point in the narrative, the animal is wounded, unable to escape, and his hunter decides to experiment on his prey, shooting bullets into its body at whim until he declares himself "shocked to find that [he] was only tormenting . . . the noble beast," and decides to move on to killing:

> I first fired six shots with the two grooved, which must have eventually proved mortal, but as yet he evinced no visible distress; after which I fired three shots at the same part with the Dutch six-pounder. Large tears now trickled from his eyes, which he slowly shut and opened; his colossal frame quivered convulsively, and, falling on his side, he expired. The tusks of this elephant were beautifully arched, and were the heaviest I had yet met with, averaging ninety pounds weight apiece.[21]

• • •

Hunters are not the only ones who make elephants cry. *Mabra elephantophila*, a moth species found in Thailand, feeds on elephant tears. Another, *Lobocraspis griseifusa*, will not wait for tears to appear; if a creature's eyeball is dry the moth will irritate it until it begins to water.[22]

• • •

I learn the word for tear-drinking: *lachryphagy*. One could speak, for instance, of the *lachryphagous* thirst of bell hooks, who, as a child, watched old men who

approached one like butterflies, moving light and beautiful, staying still for only a moment ... They were the brown-skinned men with serious faces who were the deacons of the church, the right-hand men of god. They were the men who wept when they felt his love, who wept when the preacher spoke of the good and faithful servant. They pulled wrinkled handkerchiefs out of their pockets and poured tears in them, as if they were pouring milk into a cup. She wanted to drink those tears that like milk could nourish her and help her grow.[23]

*   *   *

Milk and tears are the only bodily fluids humans can generally imagine drinking without overwhelming disgust.

*   *   *

In Turkey, on Mount Sipylus, rainwater sometimes seeps through a limestone rock formation, and people associate this "weeping rock" with the story of Niobe, who was punished for her pride in her children—neatly, mathematically, completely. She boasted that Leto had only two children to her fourteen, and so those two took revenge: Apollo killed her seven sons, Artemis her seven daughters. Her husband took his own life. Niobe herself could not stop weeping. She turned to stone, but even that could not halt her tears.

*   *   *

A fragment from Sappho tells us, "Leto and Niobe were beloved friends."[24]

*   *   *

I have no sons and no daughters. I have many beloved friends, some with one child or two.

✦ ✦ ✦

I have not wanted to approach the subject of the crying infant, because my husband, Chris, and I are trying to create one of our own, but my research keeps listing in that direction. Last night, in bed, I read of how parents in various cultures try to stop the wailing of their babies. Some tell them to stop their shouting, a command the babies eventually obey. Some shout more loudly than the baby's own cry, and then laugh until the baby is too confused or distracted or entertained to continue.[25] A colicky baby is simply a baby who cries excessively, in some cases eighteen hours a day.[26] I worry I will be a colicky mother. I worry I will not be a mother at all.

✦ ✦ ✦

I worry I will be a colicky mother because I am periodically overcome with complete, encompassing fear and despair, and when I am suffering thus, my crying can go on for hours. I rock myself on the floor and keen. I don't know why. It is one of the things my body does, like sleeping or making poems.

✦ ✦ ✦

Around this Ohio house we rented to take the job to support the existence of the imagined baby, very few cars drive by. For the first time since we adopted our cat, we feel safe letting him explore the outdoors. A few moments ago I heard him meowing to be let back inside, and when I opened the door I saw the evidence of a fight with the neighbor's cat: a scratch beginning just beneath the corner of his left eye. A red path for where a tear might run.

◆ ◆ ◆

I have begun in our new house to gather what Chris has dubbed a "crybrary." *Crying* by Tom Lutz. *Pictures & Tears* by James Elkins. The latter begins with my new favorite table of contents. I'm drawn to its gentle teasing, its naming without judgment: Chapter 1, "Crying at nothing but colors," Chapter 5, "Weeping over bluish leaves."[27]

◆ ◆ ◆

All this reading could prove a mistake. What if—to use an example from the crybrary—just as James Elkins's years of study in art history interfered with his ability to cry at paintings, my meager months of tearful research alter the way I weep at my life? Or should I be glad for the change? The summer is ending and the darkening evenings—which in other years brought me fatigue and sorrow—now close over me lightly. There have been seasons of such tears I thought myself lost. Mad. Maybe these books are a protection.

◆ ◆ ◆

Sometimes suspicion of tears—an intellectual detachment—is warranted. Consider the actor who told his friend Tom Lutz that "whenever he needed tears for a scene he conjured up a daydream to elicit them," most recently imagining "he was on the *Titanic* as it was sinking . . . and that he was handing his wife and baby son into a lifeboat."[28] Lutz, curious about the actor's explanation that "the image produced the most intense feeling of loss he could imagine,"[29] probed further, and at last his friend

> realized that the scene's effectiveness on him was based on the fact that others were watching and approving of what he was doing—the captain of the ship, the first mate, the other men taking charge of the situation. This daydream, this mini-melodrama, makes him weep because in it he consummately fulfills an iconographic social role.[30]

◆ ◆ ◆

Of course an actor's tears are purposefully generated. I know this, though I can set the knowledge aside when I watch a movie. But the artifice does not end there. It goes on, it spreads, so that even the one crying—the one to whom the tears ought to be legible—achieves at first only a super-ficial understanding. "Boy, why are you crying?" He does not know. He cannot say. And when he can, the reason is embarrassing.

◆ ◆ ◆

When one director needed the young Shirley Temple to cry for a movie scene, he told her that her mother had been "[k]idnapped by an ugly man! All green, with blood-red eyes!" Temple wept, the camera rolled. Both Temple and her mother were angry when they learned of the director's unnecessary deception, as the young performer already knew how to cry on cue, so long as the scene was filmed in the morning, before events of the day could "dilut[e her] subdued mood." "Crying," said Temple, "is too hard after lunch."[31]

◆ ◆ ◆

One afternoon the test says yes, pregnant, good job, very clever. I do not cry. Chris does not cry. I call my mother, who says, "I'm going to cry," and who does. My faithful throat lump shows up. I notice it. I begin to accept its invitation, when it occurs to me that I am fulfilling an iconographic so-cial role, and my slide into tears abruptly stops. "It's okay," I tell my mother, "It's a big deal. You're allowed to cry."

Weeks later, on a plane, a terrible tanned businessman drops a full bottle of water on my head. I'm bruised, surprised, tired, and his apology is inadequate. He does not feel bad enough. I do not want to cry, but I do, or I think I do not want to cry, but the unthinking part of me does, or perhaps, as the books say, these tears *are* a form of communication, an instruction to the man to feel worse. I summon up all my theories, trying to place them between me and the crying, trying to slow my breath with reason, but nothing helps. If I want to cry now I cannot. If I do not want to I cannot stop. Perhaps I ought to have surrendered to it, the wave of oncoming of tears. The empty seat next to me I count as a blessing.

＊ ＊ ＊

People often cry on planes. A survey of Virgin Atlantic passengers found that 41 percent of men "said they'd hidden under blankets to hide their tears," while women "reported hiding tears by pretending they had something in their eye."[32]

＊ ＊ ＊

Why planes? Perhaps it is the stillness of the ride, after all the stress of motion: you get to the airport, part from loved ones, half undress and unpack yourself through security, huff and sweat to the gate and onto the plane. The body at rest suddenly finds its feelings have caught up, and—as you've neglected them in favor of more practical concerns—they arrive loudly, demanding immediate physical expression. Or maybe it is the blankets. Online one person tells me, "i cried in the airplane when my twin sister told me i was ugliest when i smiled. i threw a blanket over my head and cried." Lately, when I get on a plane, I imagine the blanket the flight attendant hands me is still damp with the last passenger's tears.

◆   ◆   ◆

Maybe they are the tears of Mary Ruefle, the poet, who—in an essay on making poetry by erasing books—writes of a moment when she told her airplane seatmate about her work, which the woman kindly and sweetly misunderstands, and then:

> as the air of the airplane was suddenly warm and oppressive, I struggled to remove my overcoat, and when she reached out to help me I was overcome by this unexpected and tender gesture of assistance and to my great embarrassment, and for reasons having nothing to do with our conversation, I began to cry. And she said, "Don't worry, dear, God works in mysterious ways."[33]

＊ ＊ ＊

Maybe we cannot know the real reason why we are crying.
Maybe we do not cry *about*, but rather *near* or *around*. Maybe
all our explanations are stories constructed after the fact.
Not just stories. I won't say *just*.

＊ ＊ ＊

I want the act of reading these tears, of placing them alongside
one another, to make not story, but relationship emerge. This
tear and this tear and this one. I mean what Jack Spicer meant
when he wrote to Federico García Lorca, who was dead:

> I would like to make poems out of real objects.
> The lemon to be a lemon that the reader could cut
> or squeeze or taste—a real lemon like a newspa-
> per in a collage is a real newspaper. I would like
> the moon in my poems to be a real moon, one
> which could be suddenly covered with a cloud
> that has nothing to do with the poem—a moon
> utterly independent of images. The imagination
> pictures the real. I would like to point to the real,
> disclose it, to make a poem that has no sound in
> it but the pointing of a finger.[34]

A real tear that you can taste, a moon that has nothing to do
with crying. (The latter does not exist.)

* * *

Walking through Fort Greene one weekend, Bill and I found a box of free books on the sidewalk, a fantastic collection of anthologies for schoolchildren from the Penguin English Project, published in the 1970s. We flipped excitedly through the pages, delighting at the casual way the editors let poems adjoin children's conversations, let photographs brush against myth. Bill tried to convince me to take all the books for myself, but I made him keep one. A souvenir of our happy day. Years later, when Neil Armstrong died, I returned to one volume's transcript of the moon landing to make from it an elegy. I wonder where Bill's book is now, feel afraid it has been thrown away.

* * *

The baby is my first thought upon waking each morning. I sleep, I wake, with my hands over my belly. She stirs and before any other image can occur to me I flood into the moment when I will first hold her. What will I say? "I have dreamed of you so much that you are no longer real," writes Robert Desnos to his beloved, "I have dreamed of you so much that my arms, grown used to being crossed on my chest as I hugged your shadow, would perhaps not bend to the shape of your body."[35] In the dark, in the new morning, I meet my shadowy child. *You're here, you're here, it's you, hello*, and I swipe away my tears before they hit the pillow. In the dark of the ultrasound room we saw her face in black and white, her bright nose, her actual mouth. What will I say through both of our crying? And my tears, here, now in this bed, are they merely the perfunctory by-product of the iconographic scene? And why *merely*? This transformation will happen, I will become a mother, a shadow, "a hundred times more shadow than the shadow that moves and goes on moving, brightly, over the sundial of your life."[36] The weight of her, warm, on my chest.

◆ ◆ ◆

One morning, digging up weeds in the front garden, I listen to a lecture on emotion elicitation techniques: the stimuli researchers use to induce feelings in their laboratory subjects. The professor introduces a video often used to elicit happiness, and—because I am only hearing the podcast through my headphones—I can't see the woman celebrating her Olympic gold medal, but listen dutifully as I loosen the earth around another dandelion. Then the professor introduces a video that researchers have found a reliable tool for eliciting sadness. Distracted by my digging, I don't catch whether the video is documentary or fictional, and I immediately begin to worry about the boy whose small voice now reaches my ears. His father, a boxer, is dying. His father is calling for him. And when his father goes silent the boy pleads, "No! Champ! No! Champ. Is he out? Is he out? What's the matter, Champ? Champ, wake up! Wake up! Wake—wake up! Champ, wake up, Champ! Hey, don't sleep now. We got to go home. Got to go home, Champ."[37] I cannot keep up my digging. I am crying all over the soil. I mistook myself for a researcher, when I am a weeping subject.

✦ ✦ ✦

Days later I learn that the clip comes from the 1979 film *The Champ*, and I watch the death scene onscreen. This time I know I do not need to worry for an actual child, but the tears return anyhow. I'm reminded of a story by Amy Hempel that ends with the narrator recollecting what she knows of a chimp who could communicate using sign language:

> I think of the chimp, the one with the talking hands.
>
> In the course of the experiment, that chimp had a baby. Imagine how her trainers must have thrilled when the mother, without prompting, began to sign to her newborn.
>
> Baby, drink milk.
>
> Baby, play ball.

And when the baby died, the mother stood over
the body, her wrinkled hands moving with animal grace, forming again and again the words:
Baby, come hug, Baby, come hug, fluent now in
the language of grief.[38]

When I first heard this story read aloud over the radio I was
utterly unprepared for the crying it invited, and in my confused sadness, went looking for this chimp, only to find that
Hempel had fictionalized and intensified a somewhat different story. Upon learning of a caretaker's miscarriage, the real
chimp, Washoe, signed *Cry*.[39] I examine my feelings, report
to myself: *This stimulus elicits zero tears*.

◆ ◆ ◆

Someone says *tears*, and the noun triggers the expected verb:
fall. Always they fall *like rain*. These sentences, a long and
inattentive marriage. Or sometimes, less frequently, tears
land. On the page, on the face of the beloved. In space tears
neither fall nor land. In a video, an astronaut—a Canadian
with a mustache—demonstrates this by squirting drinking
water from a silver pouch into his left eye. He is not even
slightly sad. The water clings to itself, a clear glob, a large
and misshapen meniscus.[40] If a drop escapes into the air, it's
not hard to say what it does next. In space every noun mar-
ries *float*.

Besides his disappearance at sea, Bas Jan Ader, the Dutch-born performance artist, is most famous for a few short experimental films. In *I'm Too Sad to Tell You* the handwritten title appears for several seconds, and then the film cuts to Ader weeping—tears spilling from his eyes, head nodding and shaking by turn, mouth opening and closing as if to swallow his sadness—for just over three minutes. I do not know why he is crying, but when I watch I feel myself nodding with him, affirming his great sorrow.

* * *

In his series of "Fall" films, Ader slides off the roof of his house in a chair, hangs by his arms from a tree until he drops into a river, tilts sideways and falls over a sawhorse, rides his bicycle with no hesitation into a canal. Again, the films provide no reason for his actions, but elsewhere, in a brief artist's statement, Ader offers an explanation whose simplicity and clarity seem to me inarguably accurate: "When I fell off the roof of my house, or into a canal, it was because gravity made itself master over me. When I cried, it was because of extreme grief."[41]

* * *

A fall is elementary, primal, basic. It is, in the words of Anne Carson, "our earliest motion. A human is born by falling, as Homer says, from between the knees of its mother. To the ground. We fall again at the end: what starts on the ground will end up soaking into the ground forever."[42]

* * *

The events then, of a life, could be reduced to a swift symmetry: *fall, cry, fall.* If we are in the mood for reduction.

* * *

On the moon, where the astronaut Alan Shepard cried, gravity exerts one sixth of the force it does on Earth. Tears fall, but more slowly, like snow. I learned this as a child at Space Camp, where I cried because I wanted to play the role of mission specialist in our mock flight, but was assigned instead to be the public affairs officer. Mine was not to do, but to describe.

* * *

In my first version of the sentences above, I wrote that it was Buzz Aldrin who cried on the moon, but my memory failed me. Neil Armstrong also did not weep, or at least his tears did not fall. Back in the lunar module, Aldrin photographed Armstrong with wet eyes. Would tears have dropped had they been here on Earth?

◆ ◆ ◆

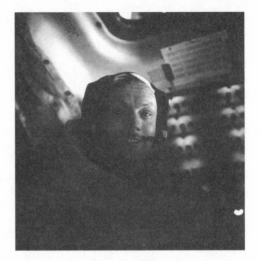

◆ ◆ ◆

Aldrin triggers *Neil Armstrong*, but *Armstrong* does not trig-
ger *Aldrin*. Theirs is an unequal marriage. After they returned to Earth, Aldrin drank his sorrows away, then two
wives. The tears behaved according to tradition, falling like
rain on the land.

◆ ◆ ◆

Today again snow falls from not that far up in the sky. Inside
me the baby is floating like a noun in space, but she can tell
which way is up, which way down.

• • •

Almost as soon as movies were invented they flew a rocket ship into the moon's eye, stimulating tears.

• • •

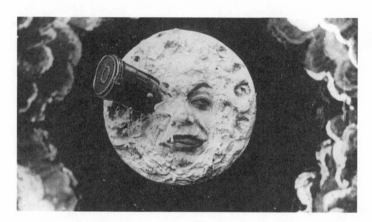

• • •

I heard a story of a young guy who used to go for walks with an older poet, a dispenser of lyrical wisdom. *Leave the moon alone*, he advised.

• • •

Paige insists this kind of advice must be ignored: "Don't trust anyone who says 'Poetry has had enough of these things.' Because what they're actually saying is 'I have had enough of these things.' & how could anyone who's 'had enough of the moon' be right about poetry?"[43]

◆ ◆ ◆

A person who "cries for the moon" wants too much—wants, in fact, more wanting—weeps into the lack. You can't make a wish upon the moon.

◆ ◆ ◆

Shirley Temple cried real tears when a classmate died, she writes in her autobiography, and they stained the page of the classmate's yearbook photo. To the official caption, "She would give you the moon if she had it," the actress made a small addition, "carefully ink[ing] one word, 'Dead.'"[44]

◆ ◆ ◆

Asked about the moon's composition in 1902, children respond:

> It is made of rags . . . or the man in it is stuffed
> with them . . . it is a picture with yellow

paint . . . made of yellow paper . . . putty . . .
gold . . . silver . . . honey . . . cotton . . . a lucky
stone . . . a cake of ice . . . of many stars . . .
air . . . brass . . . a plate . . . a balloon . . .
clouds . . . a ball . . . tallow . . . a lamp, candle
or gas . . . of light . . . of dirt . . . water . . .
cloth . . . a bundle of sticks on fire . . . milk . . .
butter . . . felt . . . lightning . . . made of dead
people who join hands in a circle of light . . .
some bright dish hung up . . . water and dirt
like the earth . . . a dead skull . . . a water
pail . . . it is God, Christ, or anyone else . . .
is the face or head of some dead relative or
friend . . . stuck through the clouds, or the
body goes straight toward the sky and is hidden from us by the head.[45]

Their collection of answers acts upon me like a spell, leaves
me enchanted, bewitched. It is a "heap of language," a pile
of moon dust. Or it is a house made entirely of windows, in
every one a child's round face.

◆ ◆ ◆

This winter, if the wood from outside the supermarket was
too damp to catch fire, we'd add Fatwood sticks from inside
the supermarket, and this is civilization, which NASA says

will come to an end in the article I won't read, because today I don't feel like crying.

✦ ✦ ✦

We don't need wood anymore. It is the first day of spring and I need daffodils, but they're not yet apparent, so instead I look at the picture my mother sent me of her mother in a whole field of them. Kew Gardens, perhaps, the park just minutes from their flat. I think of William Carlos Williams's poem "The Last Words of My English Grandmother," which ends with a journey to the hospital:

> On the way
> we passed a long row
> of elms. She looked at them
> awhile out of
> the ambulance window and said,
>
> What are all those
> fuzzy-looking things out there?
> Trees? Well, I'm tired
> of them and rolled her head away.[46]

Mr. Williams, I too had an English grandmother, but I don't know her last words, only that she died in South Africa near her older daughter, who moved there with her husband, formerly a student of gardening at Kew.

◆ ◆ ◆

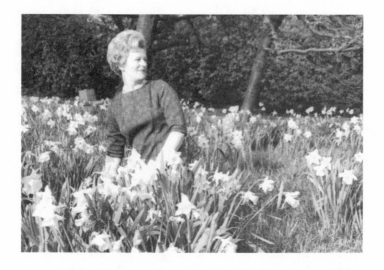

◆ ◆ ◆

We treat the dying as if they've lost their reason, as infants who've somehow misbehaved. We want them to be good. The dying want their mothers, but their mothers are nowhere to be found, are maybe still back among the flowers. How Bill died I do not understand. I mean this literally. I do not know what happened. By then we barely spoke. If I saw him at all I saw him agitated and drunk, and it was simpler to avoid his company.

◆ ◆ ◆

Who moves to South Africa in 1962? My aunt, a white English woman. Her husband, a white Dutch man. We did not visit until 1992, when Apartheid was coming at last to an end. White people seemed fitful, afraid. "I'd rather burn my house down than let them have it," said one, in his pinched accent. I remember only a single instance of crying from this trip. My sister and I, trapped, in our aunt's backyard pool. The Rottweiler—a pet or a guard dog—circled and circled, growling, would not let us out. Of the few commands he understood, my uncle most often told him to *voetsek*, Afrikaans for "fuck off." We were afraid he'd tear us in two.

◆　◆　◆

Early this morning the radio says divers have taken the first photographs of a steamship that sank in 1880, when it was split in two by another ship in heavy fog. Standing in the darkness of the kitchen I understand this as a metaphor for giving birth.

◆　◆　◆

Errol Morris's documentary about the former secretary of defense Robert McNamara, *The Fog of War*, borrows its title from a Prussian military theorist, who wrote:

> Finally, the general unreliability of all infor-
> mation presents a special problem in war: all
> action takes place, so to speak, in a kind of twi-
> light, which, like fog or moonlight, often tends

to make things seem grotesque and larger than they really are.[47]

✦ ✦ ✦

Last night the television played endless clips of crying politicians, including one misty-eyed candidate whose impending grandparenthood has pundits predicting her campaign's emotional weather.

✦ ✦ ✦

Struck by associations and without pen or paper, I run from the kitchen to search the house for what I need, and when I turn my head for a moment away from the page I've begun to scribble, I see the milk I was warming on the stove is about to boil over.

✦ ✦ ✦

When my baby is born the smell of milk will draw her slowly up to my breast. I've seen videos, the newborn inching gradually to the nipple, through the confusion of the brightest light she's ever known.

✦ ✦ ✦

People talk about the fog of pregnancy, the forgetfulness, the book neatly put away in the refrigerator. The other week

I tried to make a new friend, but became distracted before writing down my phone number's last two digits.

◆ ◆ ◆

I prefer to cry with a friend, but these days I am often alone. Exhausted by an argument with Chris, I retreat to the solitude of the bathroom.

◆ ◆ ◆

Another friend tells me that upon learning she was pregnant she thought, "I'm not alone anymore."

◆ ◆ ◆

When I am sobbing on the bathroom floor, what does the baby feel?

◆ ◆ ◆

Chris knocks on the door and we postpone the argument, but I cannot stop weeping all over the linoleum. The argument is about the cat, whether he will be allowed to sleep in the room with us, with the baby. All I can think of is the cat's own crying, which I cannot bear. People often mistake the cries of a cat for those of an infant. They say this may be a wise adaptation on the animal's part. I am crying because I am afraid of losing myself in the fog.

◆ ◆ ◆

One fog points to another. I can see in my pregnant tears the shape of those shed in other moments. This frightens me. Am I lost already? How far? How far to go?

◆ ◆ ◆

When I am in the fog of despair I fear I cry too much to be a good partner or parent or person, that something within me is utterly broken, that any reprieve—a day of joy! a poem!— is temporary and somehow false. But that is the fog doing its work, making everything large and grotesque. When the fog lifts I can point up, say *Look, it is a cloud.*

◆ ◆ ◆

One of the ways Chris loves me is that he waits while I cry. He tells me it will pass. He does not leave. And when the fog lifts he makes space for me to write.

◆ ◆ ◆

When the contractions begin, I take a shower. My hair has reached a point of greasiness that makes it difficult for me to concentrate on anything else—even giving birth—and I figure I have some time. But when I get out of the shower the contractions are just four minutes apart. Every time one hits I hand the hair dryer to my sister, who has flown out from New England along with my mother for the occasion. When the pain recedes she passes it back. Eventually I give up, wind the long strands into a bun. Days later, delivered and delirious, when I finally take my hair down again, it will still be wet.

◆ ◆ ◆

The pain is very bad. I do not shed tears. I moan. I try to find words for myself, an adequate image. *I am a giant bear riding a tiny tricycle of pain. I am a brown paper bag with no bottom and the pain is falling through me.* It does not diminish the pain, but it gives me something else to hold in my body: the satisfaction of having shaped an accurate description.

◆ ◆ ◆

After a night of vomiting with every contraction and a day of sucking popsicles through the glorious numbness of an epidural, the doctor tells me it is time for a C-section, and that—as I am at risk for massive hemorrhaging—he may have to remove my uterus along with the baby. I sink into a terrible dry calm, while my sister, who has not slept, begins to cry. I understand she is crying because she is witnessing a difficult and maybe sorrowful event. I understand I am not crying because I am the event.

• • •

The human lacrimal system develops in fetuses weeks before birth, but an infant's first cries are dry-eyed shouts. Immobile on the table, I hear the baby wail as the surgeon lifts her from my cut belly. Then he tucks my uterus back in.

• • •

Before she was born—as a kind of immersive preparation—I watched hour after hour of *One Born Every Minute*, a British reality show chronicling labor and births in a maternity ward. My mirror neurons, shiny and alert. "Poor baby, poor baby," I'd murmur, meaning the wailing mother.

• • •

Just barely I manage to read *The New York Times* on the laptop while the baby nurses. One mother, says the article, held the erroneous conviction that she had caused her baby irrevocable brain damage. The woman felt her guilt so fiercely she strapped the baby to her chest and leapt to her death. The baby—the article waits until its last sentence to tell me—survived.[48] I do not cry, because before I began I blocked feeling, told myself I would read as if purely for information.

Data. A distant story while my own baby suckles and slurps. She is not me, the baby is not my baby. Mirror neurons, those little synaptic empathy gears, I've stopped with a wrench.

✦ ✦ ✦

Empathy can be a hole through which one falls into despair. Tears make the ground slippery. And then what? Satisfaction for the depth of one's feeling? If I am not myself in danger, then my imagining myself into the place of another's suffering unnecessarily incapacitates me, makes me unable to move some small part of my day in a direction that would make other lives more possible. And at this moment, my body still working to knit itself back together, the task is not to fall apart. The task is to remain.

✦ ✦ ✦

When Margery Kempe, the English medieval mystic famous for her near-constant weeping, gave birth to her first child, she became afflicted with what we might now interpret as postpartum psychosis, and saw

> devils opening their mouths all alight with burning flames of fire, as if they would have swallowed her in, sometimes pawing at her, sometimes threatening her, sometimes pulling her and hauling her about both night and

day. [. . .] She would have killed herself many a time as they stirred her to, and would have been damned with them in hell, and in witness of this she bit her own hand so violently that the mark could be seen for the rest of her life.[49]

She was returned to her senses by a visit from Jesus Christ, who was dressed in purple silk—*like Prince!* says Gabrielle—and gazed at her "with so blessed a countenance that she was strengthened in all her spirits."[50]

✦ ✦ ✦

Once, approaching Jerusalem, Kempe's ecstatic tears grew so intense that she almost fell off her donkey.[51] I wish she could laugh at herself, but she refuses.

✦ ✦ ✦

Hers is the English language's first autobiography. We had a wet beginning!

✦ ✦ ✦

The baby is one week old and she will not stop crying. I sing "Be My Baby" to her, but the song so deeply fails to describe our circumstances that it only makes me cry as well. An hour into the noise, my mother tries to enter the bedroom to help us, but I turn her away. Then Chris, then my sister. I can see myself too clearly in their worried faces, can see the pity that I then can't help but share. If we are to stop crying, pity must not be allowed in. We close our eyes, go it alone, try to see not ourselves but each other.

✦ ✦ ✦

Almost all of my understanding is from books. My mother worries I have read too much about parenting, that I am all theory and no heart. She might be right. Sometimes it seems there are more pages in me than breaths. I know how to receive and shape and store these black words, have taken them as instructions. When I was a child I read my mother's copy of *Your Gifted Child* and made awkward attempts to perform its descriptions. Later I borrowed her *Reviving Ophelia*, a therapist's account of treating adolescent girls who experience sexual assault, eating disorders, self-harm, suicidality. We did our best to prepare.

✦ ✦ ✦

It is even through reading that I learn how Bill died, in a poem by my friend Mathias:

> I'm thinking
> of the last time I ran
> into Billy Cassidy
> in Williamsburg

& both of us were like
We should hang out soon!
but New York being
the what that it is
we knew we
probably wouldn't.

And then Jules telling me
he had killed himself
& finding this out
at the AWP Conference
& we wept
& looked at stacked books on sale
on the table for the University of California
        Press.[52]

I know that Jules must have told me too when she called me that morning and I answered the phone in the hotel bathroom, but somehow the *NOs* I uttered as I sank to the cold floor interfered with the fact of his suicide making its way into my long-term memory. It was not until Mathias's poem that I knew for certain, that I understood. I could not fathom his death through a phone, but I can fathom a book, a line.

◆ ◆ ◆

I remember the first time I met Jules, walking with Bill to go hear Rachel Zucker give a reading. It was spring, sunny, still cold. "What dark thing have you done to me?" asked one poem. "Not dark enough."[53]

◆ ◆ ◆

For the first month of her life, the baby receives her dreams through the mail, one a day, slipped inside a pink #10 envelope. We have signed her up for Mathias's dream delivery service. "You are holding on to a rope that goes up into the sky," he writes. "You are floating in a basket in a river." "You are playing chess against the Dalai Lama & you have a suspicion that he is letting you win." For June 30, the last day, he writes:

You are looking in a mirror, but the baby in the mirror does not do what you do. When you move your arm the baby in the mirror does not move its arm. Instead it moves its head. When you move your head the baby in the mirror opens its mouth. Inside its mouth there is a fishbowl & some fishes are swimming around in circles. This makes you laugh. You know that when you grow up you will be filled with fishes & they will make you happy & strong.

When he and Jules were still a couple Mathias made a noose with which to hang himself. Each pink envelope means he did not.

52

HEATHER CHRISTLE

They say perhaps we cry when language fails, when words can no longer adequately convey our hurt. When my crying is not wordless enough I beat my head with my fists.

+ + +

Once, when I was fourteen, I became very drunk on vodka. When my mother found and scolded me I broke a window with my head. My father was at sea. My mother called the police.

+ + +

Before they arrived, before they took me to the hospital, I half undressed myself and climbed into the bath, crying, chanting, keening, *I want to die, I want to die*. It is a song my body knows.

+ + +

And I do not know whether the song comes from within or without, whether it is called forward by structures in the world or structures in my blood. Both, and, neither, all. It is a song with so few words. Subject verb infinitive. I keep it there, unconjugated.

♦ ♦ ♦

In college, in Deborah Digges's class on poets in exile, Sylvia Plath consumed one quarter of our attention. In discussions Deborah sounded preoccupied with sympathy for the poet as a struggling young mother. I remember the feeling of Plath's various identities suddenly aligning in my head like an eclipse. I don't know which one was the sun, which the moon. *The moon is no door. It is a face in its own right.*[54] Of the four poets we read together—Plath, Marina Tsvetaeva, Anna Akhmatova, María Elena Cruz Varela—two killed themselves. Akhmatova died of heart failure. Varela is still alive. On April 10, 2009, Deborah died after jumping from a stadium at the University of Massachusetts, near her home in Amherst.

♦ ♦ ♦

I remember one class where we discussed Sylvia Plath's "Tulips," a poem I love, in which the titular flowers (a gift during a hospital stay) undergo a series of dramatic metaphorical transformations, restlessly shifting through images as the poet's mind reimagines both the flowers and her own body. And I remember Deborah posing a question at some point, asking whether any of us thought she was overreacting to the flowers. "They're just *tulips*, Sylvia," she said, trying out the idea.

* * *

Last Christmas, my sister gave her fiancé a copy of *A Pattern Language*, a guide to building houses, neighborhoods, towns, communities. In a section titled "The Poetry of the Language" I read:

> It is possible to make buildings by stringing together patterns, in a rather loose way. A building made like this, is an assembly of patterns. It is not dense. It is not profound. But it is also possible to put patterns together in such a way that many many patterns overlap in the same physical space: the building is very dense; it has many meanings captured in a small space and through this density, it becomes profound.[55]

* * *

It seems a strange choice, to die at the stadium. In a poem beginning with this thought and then descending elsewhere, Lisa writes "I would have / chosen the bridge."[56] A bridge is profound, dense with its connections. So dense, perhaps, that it is more metaphor than structure. John Berryman leapt from a metaphor and perished. Hart Crane, author of his own *Bridge*, chose not to end his life there, elected instead to slip from a ship to the sea. James Baldwin walked the bridge and turned back.[57] A bridge, like the moon, is several. *The moon is my mother. I have fallen a long way.*[58] But the stadium. The stadium feels like prose, like information.

◆ ◆ ◆

I am making a sandwich in the kitchen when the radio tells me that in the town next to ours, police have shot and killed John Crawford III, a young black man walking through Walmart, carrying a toy gun he'd picked from a store shelf. "No, no, no," I say, I cry out. To whom? The baby is asleep. The radio can't hear me. It is telling me the weather.

◆ ◆ ◆

The scholar Christina Sharpe, author of *In the Wake: On Blackness and Being*, says that "in [her] text, the weather is the totality of our environments; the weather is the total climate; and that climate is antiblack."[59] She was my teacher too; I go on learning. The day that a grand jury fails to indict two police officers for killing Tamir Rice, Ashley C. Ford writes, "You should know a 12 year-old boy's murder has been chalked up to 'a perfect storm of human error' and you should wonder about the weather."[60]

◆ ◆ ◆

"White tears" are tears shed by a white person who has been made suddenly aware of systemic racism, or her own implication within white supremacy. They can be a form of defense against an imagined aggression, a way of shutting down a conversation the white person finds hurtful. "Are you calling me a *racist?*!" Commence weeping. Brittney Cooper explains the particular power of tears at the intersection of whiteness and femininity:

> White-lady tears might seem not to be a big deal, but they are actually quite dangerous. When white women signal through their tears that they feel unsafe, misunderstood, or attacked, the whole world rises in their defense. The mythic nature of white female vulnerability compels protective impulses to arise in all men, regardless of race.[61]

✦ ✦ ✦

I do not want to redeem those tears. I want to read them for what they are and I want to read beyond them. But they are heavy, heavy in the weather.

✦ ✦ ✦

When Ronald Ritchie—the white man whose white wife prompted him to call 911 on John Crawford—described the scene at Walmart to the operator, he lied that Crawford had pointed the toy gun at a couple of children. In the surveillance video, you can see the children and their mother—a white woman named Angela Williams—shopping unconcernedly near Crawford. When the police arrived and shot Crawford, Williams ran in fear with her children, suffered a heart attack, and died. In the name of the protection of mythic white femininity, police killed a black man and the white woman they imagined he would make weep.[62]

◆   ◆   ◆

Here is another way to say it. Because people like the Ritchies can look at a woman and child with skin like mine, and see our bodies as full of tears on the verge of being spilled, they can talk themselves into seeing real bullets in a toy gun. They can make of us an occasion—a weather event—on which they are permitted to call forth death.

◆   ◆   ◆

In 1908, Alvin Borgquist, a white graduate student at Clark University in Massachusetts, published the first in-depth psychological study on crying. Gathering data for his work, he created a questionnaire for respondents to fill out, whose instructions began:

Describe a cry with utter abandon. Did it bring a sense of utter despair? Describe as fully as you can such an experience in yourself, your subjective feelings, how it grew, what caused and increased it, its physical symptoms, and all its aftereffects. What is wanted is a picture of a genuine and unforced fit or crisis of pure misery.[63]

✦ ✦ ✦

Borgquist sent his survey to schools around the United States, receiving returns from "161 females and 39 males."[64] I imagine—as he felt no need to mark their race—that the respondents were white. In his explanation of source materials, he wrote that it "has been extensively supplemented by ethnological data secured, for the most part, through the Bureau of American Ethnology, and its reports and from the Archives of Aboriginal Knowledge."[65] He also wrote to W. E. B. Du Bois, not to ask the questions he asked in his standard survey, but rather to say:

> Dear Sir:
>
> We are forming an investigation here on the subject of crying as an expression of the emotions, and should like very much to learn about its peculiarities among the colored people. We have been referred to you as a person competent to give us information upon the subject.
>
> We desire especially to know about the following salient aspects.
>
> 1. Whether the negro sheds tears.[66]

＊ ＊ ＊

When Lucille Clifton learned of Borgquist's question she composed her own "reply":

> he do
> she do
> they live
> they love
> they try
> they tire
> they flee
> they fight
> they bleed
> they break
> they moan
> they mourn
> they weep
> they die
> they do
> they do
> they do[67]

＊ ＊ ＊

For a moment Clifton considered shifting that last "they" to "we," but decided against it.[68] She left no record of why she made that decision, but the choice engenders in me a sense of the speaker's exhausted question to the white audience: *How many times must you be told?*

*   *   *

What is it like to photograph crying? To fight the urge to intervene and replace it with the urge to document? Charles Darwin wrote, "It is easy to observe infants while screaming; but I have found photographs made by the instantaneous process the best means for observation, as allowing more deliberation,"[69] and so he relied, at times, on other people's images. Still, he found many occasions to observe the tears and screams of his own offspring:

> Infants whilst young do not shed tears or weep, as is well known to nurses and medical men. This circumstance is not exclusively due to the lacrymal glands being as yet incapable of secreting tears. I first noticed this fact from having accidentally brushed with the cuff of my coat the open eye of one of my infants, when seventy-seven days old, causing this eye to water freely; and though the child screamed violently, the other eye remained dry, or was only slightly suffused with tears.[70]

*   *   *

The baby sheds her first tears at the doctor's office, following her three-month vaccination shots. I put her to my breast to nurse and stare at her streaked cheeks, wondering how I might preserve the moment, how I might save those tears. I kiss them away, write it down.

❖ ❖ ❖

At home when the baby is crying I have no thoughts but how to console her. Language leaves me. "Go away," I tell Chris. "Fuck you," I tell him. The only words I can muster.

❖ ❖ ❖

At the end of the week, on my birthday, I will fly down to Florida with the baby for my American grandmother's funeral. Last night I wrote a list of what to pack: the rubber giraffe, a sun hat, waterproof mascara. This will be the baby's first time to see the ocean.

❖ ❖ ❖

It was when fish became terrestrial amphibians that the body's lacrimal system first evolved.[71] We left the water and began to weep the home we'd abandoned.

❖ ❖ ❖

My father, the merchant mariner, no longer goes to sea. In his new retirement he is busy tending to the garden. Before, crossing from California to Japan, he would navigate the giant container ship away from the Great Pacific Ocean Garbage Patch. Fish do not, *cannot*, cry.

◆ ◆ ◆

At the funeral I do not see my father cry. The priest, whose clip-on microphone sputters in and out, riffs on his digital woes for several minutes, before a graceless segue to the subject of my dead grandmother: "But Margaret doesn't have to worry about technical difficulties anymore." When he invites her children each to share a specific memory of her, they respond with blank generalizations: she loved her family, she worked very hard. At the reception, in a bland community room, our little node of the family—my father, mother, sister, daughter, and I—sit together around one table. My sister, red and tired, cries that we do not really know our aunts and uncles, that we had shown our love for our grandmother poorly. We eat cold bagels. Someone asks my sister—a former Peace Corps volunteer—with grave concern what is to be done about "the people in Africa." I am wearing a black dress with vertical zippers over the breasts, so the baby can nurse discreetly. The slender pull-tabs dangle and shine like nipple tassels on an inept stripper.

◆ ◆ ◆

In our shared memory, my sister and I can find just one time we saw our father cry, only I do not really remember it anymore. Instead I remember the story my sister wrote about it:

> I cut his hair. I get my left and right confused and cut the hair behind his ear too short. I explain his options. "Dad, I'm sorry. I'm afraid there's been a bit of an accident." He doesn't turn around. "I can either cut it all really short or I can do the same thing on the other side. What would you like me to do?" He won't get up and look in the mirror. I bring him a hand mirror and he still won't look. He asks me if I read the instructions. I tell him I read the instructions. "You wouldn't let me start until I read them." He stares straight ahead at the refrigerator. "I don't care what you did," he commands, "just fix it." He won't look at me. I set the buzzers down on the counter and move away from him in his chair in the middle of the kitchen floor. I move into the corner. I am crying. Heather gets in the corner. My dad approaches the corner. We are all in a corner and we all cry.[72]

✦ ✦ ✦

A kitchen is the best—I mean the saddest—room for tears. A bedroom is too easy, a bathroom too private, a living room too formal. If someone falls to pieces in the kitchen, in the space of work and nourishment, they must be truly coming undone. The bright lights offer no comfort, only illuminate. The floor should be vinyl and cold.

◆ ◆ ◆

Charlotte Perkins Gilman—feminist, writer, sufferer of postpartum and other depressions—proposed in 1898 that private kitchens be abolished, as the work they demanded of women left them with no time for any other activities. "The cleaning required in each house would be much reduced," she argues, "by the removal of the two chief elements of household dirt,—grease and ashes."[73] She does not mention a corresponding reduction in tears.

◆ ◆ ◆

Some churches have designated "crying rooms," soundproofed spaces to which parents of wailing infants can retreat if they are concerned about bothering their fellow parishioners. Often the room will have a large window, so that its inhabitants can still look out upon the nave and chancel, as well as speakers, so they can hear the sound of the sermon and hymns. People unfamiliar with the practice—guests, for instance, at a wedding or funeral— sometimes, understandably, mistake its purpose. The poets I know who have made this mistake are without exception very taken with the idea.

Crying rooms appear most frequently in Catholic churches. One man tells me his story of seeking forgiveness for his sins during Confession in a crying room. Not ever having made a serious confession before, and in a great deal of anguish—he was suffering the aftereffects of divorce and mental illness—the man decided to lay bare his soul, but the priest responded with what felt like a cold, detached script: a rote recommendation to turn to Christ. Unheard, unheeded, the man ran crying from the crying room.

✦ ✦ ✦

Margery Kempe's madness, or bedevilment, or suffering, was caused not only by the birth of her first child, but also—like this man's—by a priest's failure to hear her confession. She never, in her book, utters precisely the nature of her sin, only that it weighed on her terribly, and that "the devil said in her mind that she should be damned, for she was not shriven of that fault."[74] And so, when after childbirth she feared for her life, she called for her confessor, but "when she came to the point of saying that thing which she had so long concealed, her confessor was a little too hasty and began sharply to reprove her before she had fully said what she meant."[75] In consequence, "because of the dread she had of damnation on the one hand, and his sharp reproving of her on the other, this creature went out of her mind and was amazingly disturbed and tormented with spirits."[76]

* * *

Sometimes I am afraid that as I am listening to people's stories of tears—and therefore, frequently, of suffering—I will make the mistake of these priests, that I will fail to hear what people most want to be known, that I will only make them cry again.

* * *

In April 1975, five years after creating *I'm Too Sad to Tell You*, Bas Jan Ader introduced a new work in a cycle called *In Search of the Miraculous*. Conceived as a three-part project, the first installment consisted of photographs of Ader walking through Los Angeles at night, seeking something with the aid of a flashlight. For the second installment, Ader planned to sail across the Atlantic Ocean in a small sailboat by himself, having been seen off by a group of his art students singing sea shanties. The third installment was to be another series of night-wandering photographs, this time in Amsterdam, but Ader disappeared during his sea voyage, and so the final piece of the triptych remains potential, conceptual, unexecuted.[77]

Three months after Bas Jan Ader set sail in his boat, his mother wrote a poem:

> I feel my heart beating too. It will go on beating
>   for some time. Then it will stop.
> I wonder if the little heart that has beaten with
>   mine, has stopped.
> When he passed the border of birth, I laid him
>   at my breast,
> Rocked him in my arms.
> He was very small then.
>
> A white body of a man, rocked in the arms of
>   the waves,
> Is very small too.[78]

A particular cruelty to losing someone to disappearance at sea is the uncertainty of knowing when the tears ought to begin. Today? Long ago? There is a mist.

✦ ✦ ✦

In 1991, when our neighbors were tying yellow ribbons around everything they owned, my father worked on an oil tanker, the only civilian ship that remained in the Persian Gulf. During the six months he was gone my mother, my sister, and I would watch the nightly news, a black screen with green dots representing missiles diverted "harmlessly out to sea." I remember one day walking into the dining room and finding my sister on my mother's lap, both of them in tears. Nothing was wrong. I mean, nothing new was wrong, I mean the war was entirely wrong, and within it my father remained safe, but the worry and the waiting had worn them down. My mother offered me her arm, invited me to join their embrace, but I shook my head. We couldn't *all* cry, I reasoned.

✦ ✦ ✦

I imagined us into a triangle, each of us nestled in her own corner. It had to be isosceles. Scalene was too erratic, equilateral too composed. I could trust neither. I am pretending this is in past tense, but honestly the feeling remains. I couldn't cry, because I needed to be the angle of difference, the angle that made the whole just unbalanced enough to keep going.

✦ ✦ ✦

But we have come all this way, and I have not explained how to cry in the first place! If you find it hard to start, Julio Cortázar's "Instructions on How to Cry" suggests picturing "a duck covered with ants," or certain bodies of water "*into which no one sails ever.*"[79]

*   *   *

In my imagination Cortázar and Ader's afterlife has them seated facing each other in a small boat, courteously taking turns practicing proper crying behavior until neither can keep a straight face, and they fill the sea air with laughter.

*   *   *

Crying won't make you feel better. We only think that it will, or, perhaps more important, think that at some point in the past it did. *Let it out*, we hear some imaginary figure instruct, and tearfully we obey. But when subjects report their mood immediately after a crying episode, it's often worse than before. Then again, this may be because the subjects are crying in a laboratory, the tears are meant to solicit aid, and the researchers provide little comfort to those whose tears they've provoked.[80]

*   *   *

Rachel disagrees, says crying for her provides a great release. She also says the half-moon looks like a taco, which makes me trust her capacity for both truth and joy.

*   *   *

It's June, and Chris and I are supposed to go teach at a writer's institute in Massachusetts, but the baby—now a full year old—has a terrible ear infection, and I have to stay home with her in Ohio. Chris goes alone. I cry at the loss of precious time with dear friends, at the chance to be someone and something other than mother. Chris is supposed to give a reading with Jim, our old teacher, our beloved poet, husband to Dara, a parent to Emily and Guy. Chris comes home. Jim dies. I turn, as one does, to his poems:

> You cannot weep;
> I cannot do anything
> that once held an ounce
> of meaning for us.
> I cover you
> with pine needles.

> When morning comes
> I will build a cathedral
> around our bodies.
> And the crickets,
> who sing with their knees,
> will come there
> in the night to be sad,
> when they can sing no more.[81]

◆ ◆ ◆

Emily and I exchange techniques to stop crying. There comes a time, we say, when one is simply not in the mood. Pick a color, she tells me, and find every instance of it in the room. I pick blue. I pick dark green. One day I call her and say that if I start to cry I want her to squawk like a chicken. When my voice starts to shake she panics and quacks like a duck. Then I am laughing and crying all at once—wet and loud and thankful—and it feels as if my heart has turned itself inside out.

◆ ◆ ◆

There are other ways to stop. One day, reading Joan Didion, I learn a new method:

> It was once suggested to me that, as an antidote to crying, I put my head in a paper bag. As it happens, there is a sound physiological reason, something to do with oxygen, for doing exactly that, but the psychological effect alone is incalculable: it is difficult in the extreme to continue fancying oneself Cathy in *Wuthering Heights* with one's head in a Food Fair bag.[82]

◆ ◆ ◆

Among wikiHow's "How to Stop Yourself from Crying," my favorite step is "Remove the lump from your throat."[83] A surgery by act of will. I imagine it falling into my hand like a doll's pacifier.

If you cannot stop your tears, or if you must take your cried-out face into public, you can hide behind a lie about allergies or a cold. You could, like Roland Barthes, don dark sunglasses:

> The intention of this gesture is a calculated one: I want to keep the moral advantage of stoicism, of "dignity" (I take myself for Clotilde de Vaux), and at the same time, contradictorily, I want to provoke the tender question ("But what's the matter with you?").[84]

• • •

I fear the tender question, whose ever-elusive answer will only stimulate more tears. The hiding is a way to stop other people from trying to help. A way to not have to explain precisely how and why I cannot be helped. I'd like to hang a little sign on each lens: *out of order*.

• • •

When Gabrielle sends me a passage from Michelle Tea's novel *Black Wave*, she is trying to help me with my writing, not with my crying, but I find ideas in it to try out in my own life:

She kept tablespoons in the freezer, would place
their rounded bottoms on her eyelids . . . She
kept chamomile tea bags soaking in the fridge.
She kept cucumbers handy and would layer her
face in slices. At a beauty store she selected a
product with raspberry extract that promised to
reduce eye puffiness.[85]

In the novel, Michelle does not find people's suggestion to
use Preparation H on puffy eyes useful, but I buy some anyway. The ointment form is too greasy, but the cream seems
to help.

✦ ✦ ✦

I love the way people offer these remedies to one another,
the care of tending, the way they try to offer an answer to
a problem without lobbing a query of their own. People
want to know: "Can the phoenix's tears bring someone
back to life?" They go to Yahoo! Answers and everyone
weighs in:

No they can only heal wounds they would not
even heal a dead persons wounds for the tears
only make the skin heal faster and dead skin
does not heal and even if it did heal the tears
cannot bring them back to life by shocking their
heart back into motion[86]

Reading this is like riding a waterslide of tears. I go down it again and again. There is no phoenix, and no phoenix tears, and nothing can bring back the dead, but these words—these hopes and these breathless responses—they *can* shock a heart back into motion. I have felt it. Have felt myself alive.

◆ ◆ ◆

Sometimes people writing answers to questions about crying will sprinkle expressions of laughter in their response.

> Q: can crying too much be dangerous ?
>
> A: it might give you a headache lol.
>
> i once had a friend who couldnt cry because her tearduct was not opened up. LOL. but when she was a little older, they got it surgically opened. haha[87]

It puzzles and charms me. It is like falling down for no reason. Or it is like finding a bruise you can't remember acquiring. Look! Poke. Poke.

◆ ◆ ◆

A doctor on YouTube points to a textbook image illustrating different parts of the lacrimal apparatus as he explains how to surgically open a blocked tear duct. The gland that produces the tears is a small blue cloud above the eye. It is raining diagonal tears. Then the doctor uses his fingers to stretch open the corner of a patient's eye, pointing out the stent he's inserted, which he describes as looking "like a little piece of spaghetti." This is the end of the explanation. Over the credits he has chosen to play "Ave Maria."

◆ ◆ ◆

Physicians have operated on the lacrimal apparatus for millennia. Restitution for botched lacrimal surgeries are even mentioned in the Code of Hammurabi. It cost more to repay a free man for the loss of his eye than an enslaved one.

◆ ◆ ◆

When Hammurabi begins a missive, he starts with a command: "To Sin-iddinam say, thus saith Hammurabi."[88] To whom is he speaking? To the person who would read the words aloud to Sin-iddinam? To the tablet itself? Written language? How surprising, this concern that the medium would need instructions for its own use. It is like explaining sorrow to tears.

◆ ◆ ◆

I love to find small stains in used books, wondering which ones originate in the lacrimal glands of weepy readers.

* * *

In the library book I've just borrowed, I see no evidence of tears, but a stranger's huge eyelash makes one whole tercet parenthetical: "so I assumed there would be, at some point, / a door with a glittering knob, / but when this would happen and where I had no idea."[89]

* * *

Stanzas are rooms, they say. A paragraph, too? I look for the doors. There is very little time. Mostly there is winter and long nights and snow.

* * *

My therapist gently proposes a diagnosis, which she further softens by questioning the idea of diagnosis in general. *Cyclothymia*. Not full-blown bipolar disorder, but adjacent. Milder, but chronic. I google it at home and read "bipolar lite." A website gathers a list of possible cyclothymes, suggests Virginia Woolf may have been one, Plath too. So that could be company, if in the afterlife they hold a convention.

* * *

Is this what made my mother so sad that winter day? Is she on the list? Have they already written my baby's name?

When people do not have a killing ability within themselves they ask gravity to do the work instead. Gravity lives in rocks. People fill the bag with rocks and kittens. Or if you are Virginia Woolf it is rocks in your pockets. I wonder if she thought *rocks* or *stones*.

. . .

Or we could try, for a while, like Hart Crane, to

> . . . make our meek adjustments,
> Contented with such random consolations
> As the wind deposits
> In slithered and too ample pockets.
>
> For we can still love the world, who find
> A famished kitten on the step . . .[90]

And I do, I try. I love the world, try to catch its tune and sing along.

. . .

It was not raining this morning when a person put an assortment of VHS exercise tapes in a cardboard box, wrote FREE on the side, and put it out on their lawn. But now it is evening, and the day was wet, and if someone tried to pick up the box now it would softly give way; the tapes would clatter and thud to the ground. That is me—not the person, the box—I have spent the day in tears. I will try to pick up an onion but it will not agree to stay in my hand. I am not going to be able to perform the acts known as *making dinner* because I am *in despair.*

+ + +

I say *despair* because it is a word that can live comfortably in a house without changing the building's purpose. It only changes the mood. *Depression* and *suicidal ideation* and *anxiety* all cast a staged or laboratory light. Even here, in this room. It shifts from paragraph to clinic.

+ + +

Despair recognizes its own ridiculousness, its emotional exaggeration. It invites you to say, like Anne of Green Gables, that you are in "the depths of despair." It makes no space for shallows.

+ + +

The *-spair* stems from the Latin for "hope." *De-* can indicate privation, reversal, or intensity, as when it doubles in on itself and *deprives.*

My despair is stupid and greedy. It wants my life but I will not give it my life, so it bargains. *Give me a finger*, it says. My despair wants me to cut off my little finger, and it wants me to use the small knife with the red handle, made by Tupperware. That is how stupid my despair is.

· · ·

It is especially hard to witness a person crying naked, like Frank O'Hara "standing in the bathtub / crying. Mother, mother / who am I?"[91] Crying is its own nakedness and to see both kinds at once elicits a panic of pity. This is why people offer handkerchiefs to each other; it is an act of care, a restoration of dignity, a small instruction to get dressed.

· · ·

If you have the money for it, you can rent, in Japan, a handsome man to wipe away your tears.[92] And you can rent a hotel room designed especially for crying.[93] There are days when it feels like happiness is a man I am renting for a fee I can no longer pay.

· · ·

I sometimes imagine a metaphysical strainer I could rinse my body through, until I am whole and clean in the sink,

and all the despair is held separate and dripping above. I
imagine I could toss it away.

I believe in ending sentences with a preposition in order to
give the ideas a way out.

+ + +

Franck André Jamme wrote his *New Exercises* on a bathroom
mirror, and in the infinitive, leaving—as did the Romans—
no space between each word, the better to obscure his face:

TOBE
ABLE
TOAL
SODI
SOBE
YANY
THOU
GHT[94]

+ + +

Carl Phillips took to the infinitive too to compose his "Gold
Leaf," which moves me—as does a mirror—simultaneously
forward and within, in this case through and back from an

animal skull held up to a face, as a way "to know utterly what you'll never be, to understand in doing so / what you are, and say no to it, not to who you are, to say no to despair."[95] Could I? Despair wants me not to know the difference between itself and me. It is a kind of decomposition. When we want someone to stop crying and we are a stern governess with one recalcitrant pupil we instruct them, *Compose yourself.*

+ + +

And what shall we make ourselves from today? A memory, a seedling, a word? What can we hold up to the light and find despair has not yet touched?

+ + +

I am teaching a beginning creative writing class and we are discussing Lorrie Moore's "People Like That Are the Only People Here," the story of a woman—a writer rather like Moore—whose baby has cancer. We go around the room, each student reading aloud the passage they found most moving and memorable, the one that brought them closest to tears.

> It is a horror and a miracle to see him. He is lying in his crib, tubed up, splayed like a boy on a

cross, his arms stiffened into cardboard "no-no"s so that he cannot yank out the tubes.

[...]

Groggy, on a morphine drip, still he is able to look at her when, maneuvering through all the vinyl wiring, she leans to hold him, and when she does he begins to cry, but cry silently, without motion or noise. She has never seen a baby cry without motion or noise. It is the crying of an old person: silent, beyond opinion, shattered.[96]

The mother cannot pick up the baby, trapped as he is in his tubes and wires. She can only lean down toward him and sing. I am so tired. My baby still does not sleep. I would like to go home and cry. What can I teach them? "Look," I tell the students. "Look at how much sadness you can make from showing sadness restrained."

◆ ◆ ◆

Clicking through images of the *pietà*—which depict Mary grieving over the body of Christ—I stumble across the "Lamentation of the Virgin" from the *Rohan Hours*, a late-medieval illuminated manuscript. Christ lies prostrate on the ground, blood marking his wounds, gray lids closed over his eyes. Mary leans desperately over him, but John the Apostle, whose own eyes are cast heavenward, clasps his arms around her torso, restraining her. She cannot reach, cannot console. I would like to punch John in his upturned face.

◆ ◆ ◆

In some versions of the *pietà*, medieval artists rendered Christ's adult body the size of a child, perhaps inspired by German mystics who wrote of Mary, in her grief, holding her dead son and imagining him a baby again. Somewhere I read that when a child dies a father will grieve its lost future and all the promise of adulthood, while a mother will grieve for her lost infant. But these are tendencies only. People tend to their dead, to their grief. Tend, tend, tender. I do not want to mistake one story, one word, for another.

◆ ◆ ◆

Last night I asked a radio reporter about his day. He'd spent it at a prison, with a group of incarcerated women who had participated in a class on producing radio stories, by and about themselves. The stories they chose to tell were heavy, said the reporter, no surprise. Yesterday they gathered to listen to the results. If the woman whose story was playing began to cry, others would join her. If the woman remained dry-eyed, so would the others, no matter how hard her tale. *There was an understanding*, said the reporter, speaking in the voice of the group, *that if she went there, we would go there with her. If she did not, neither would we.* It would be unkind to cry out of pity, to let fall from pity's vantage hurtful, unasked-for tears.

✦ ✦ ✦

Famously, the shortest sentence in the King James Bible is Mark 11:35: "Jesus wept." Other translations are somewhat less economical: "Jesus burst into tears," "And the tears of Yeshua were coming." Why did he cry? Because Lazarus, a man he loved, had died. No matter, Jesus brought him back to life.

✦ ✦ ✦

But it was speech, not tears, that resurrected the man. It was Jesus's prayer to God, and then his loud command, "Lazarus, come forth." I think of that boy in *The Champ*. "Hey, don't sleep now, Lazarus. Lazarus, wake up."

✦ ✦ ✦

The baby—my baby—is nearly two. She speaks now, in sentences, though tears still form a large part of her vocabulary. And mine. Crying is my spare room. Winter's brief suns and the ongoing sleeplessness make me a frequent visitor. Most days I cry more than I write about crying. First that strikes me as sad, but then—as if fashioning a life vest from an iceberg—I decide it strikes me as funny.

After a woman named Sarah Weed died in childbirth in New York in 1851, her husband commissioned a memorial statue of a young woman clasping a bottle to her face. It was meant to represent a tear bottle, a *lachrymatory*, a receptacle into which a mourner could let fall her hot tears, but before long a disreputable pocket magazine published a story that described the memorial as a warning against the dangers of drink, the vessel a bottle of rum.[97]

* * *

Later, a handbook for the Albany Rural Cemetery would call the magazine's story one of "many ridiculous notions" about the memorial, though its author admitted that beyond a belief that the statue is in fact intended to "illustrate some Scriptural idea," he had been unable to discover anything further.[98] Perhaps he was thinking of Psalm 56:8, an address to God that pleads, "Thou tellest my wanderings: put thou my tears into thy bottle: are they not in thy book?"

* * *

I have been wanting to write about Sarah Weed and her babe for ages, have mulled over her short life and ongoing tears, but it had not—until this morning—occurred to me that Albany is also where Bill was buried. Before long I can see the two rest in adjoining cemeteries, perhaps no more than a mile from one grave to the next.

✦ ✦ ✦

Friends keep sending me links to Rose-Lynn Fisher's photography project "The Topography of Tears." It's a series of photographs of dried tears taken through a microscope, the salt crystals forming little emotional terrains. The tears of grief blaze stark and mostly perpendicular, breaking here and there into clusters of curves. Onion tears are a dense and fernlike wallpaper. You could imagine it hanging in the house of a depthless decorator.

✦ ✦ ✦

I suspect that stories about these tears go viral because people like to see a visual—and *scientific*—depiction of the emotional range they have themselves experienced in crying. In this case, however, the science and the art only echo each other. The representation is indirect. The body makes three kinds of tears: *basal*, which are omnipresent and act as a lubricant; *irritant*, which are produced when the eye needs to be flushed of a foreign substance; and *psychogenic*, which are produced in expression of emotions. The consistent difference between psychogenic tears of grief and irritant onion tears exists not at the larger structural point of crystals, but rather the deeper layer of proteins. All psychogenic tears have higher protein levels than irritant or basal tears. Fisher herself has said that the images are dependent on much besides the emotional cause for the tears: "There are so many variables—there's the chemistry, the viscosity, the setting, the evaporation rate and the settings of the microscope." And, responding to the conversation following broad coverage of her work, she's written on her website that she's "not making any scientific claims . . . nor any declarations about anything except perhaps the poetry of life."[99]

+ + +

The baby is too old for me to call her a baby anymore. Still, she nurses, and I fantasize about our post-weaning life. My mother tells me that she still had milk even years after weaning. She tells me that early on, if she were out shopping and heard a baby cry, her milk would suddenly let down, and she'd find her shirt wet with sympathy.

+ + +

Alvin Borgquist, the man who authored the first study of crying, conducted his work under the guidance of G. Stanley Hall, then president of Clark University and the founder of the *American Journal of Psychology*. Among his other work, Hall was the co-author of "A Study of Dolls," a strange and wrenching paper, where I read:

When three, M. was given a doll, which she cher-
ished till arms, legs, and hair were gone, and it was
a painful sight, [. . .] her mother burned it; though
she had plenty of others far prettier, she cried all
night and almost all day. Her intense grief lasted
a week. Three years afterward I asked her where
Alice was; she began to cry and said: "Why did
you burn it, I loved it so, and she loved me. She is in
God's house and sometime I will see her."[100]

I am surprised to look down and see my right nipple has begun to leak.

✦ ✦ ✦

Elsewhere in the study the researchers summarize their
respondents' activities regarding the "death, funeral, and
burials of dolls":

90 children mentioned burial, their average age
being nine;

80 mentioned funerals,

73 imagined their dolls dead,

30 dug up dolls after burial to see if they had
gone to Heaven, or simply to get them back.

Of these, 11 dug them up the same day.

Only 9 speak of them as dying naturally of definitive diseases.

15 put them under sofa, in drawers, attics or gave them away, calling this death;

30 express positive belief in future life of dolls,

8 mentioned future life for them without revealing their own convictions,

3 buried dolls with pets and left them,

3 bad or dirty dolls went to the bad place,

14 to Heaven;

17 children were especially fond of funerals.

12 dolls came to accidental death by bumps or fractures,

1 burst,

1 died of a melted face,

2 were drowned (1 a paper doll),

1 died because her crying apparatus was broken,

1 doll murdered another, was tried and hung.

Dolls of which children tire often die.

30 children never imagined dolls dead. This parents often forbid.

1 boy killed his sister's doll with a toy cannon,

3 resurrected dolls and got new names,

5 out of 7 preachers at dolls' funerals were boys, 1 was the doctor.

3 doll undertakers are described.

22 cases report grief that seems to be very real and deep; in 23 cases this seemed feigned.

The mourning is sometimes real black and sometimes pretended.

19 put flowers on dolls' graves, one "all that week";

28 expressly say that dolls have no souls, are not alive, and have no future life.

In 21 cases there was death but no burial; in 10, funerals but no burials; in 8, funerals but no deaths.[101]

✦ ✦ ✦

No sound but the pointing of a finger.

✦ ✦ ✦

In Japan, people sometimes bring dolls they no longer want or need to a *ningyō kuyō*, a Buddhist or Shinto memorial ceremony, after which the dolls are burned, or in some cases recycled. There are *kuyō* ceremonies for other inanimate objects as well: eyeglasses, calligraphy brushes, chopsticks, combs, clocks, needles, knives, shoes, scissors, and semiconductors.[102]

✦ ✦ ✦

I can never quite make up my mind whether I ought to be buried or cremated. I don't want my body to rot, but I do like visitors. Company. And I am terrified of fire. As a child I often dreamt our house was burning. Sometimes I was able to rescue my most beloved doll, Carol, from the flames. Sometimes she perished.

Some nights, before I fell asleep, I'd become frightened that goblins were going to come kidnap Carol in the dark, so I'd set her way down at the foot of the bed as if she meant nothing to me. I reasoned that if the goblins believed I didn't love her, they would think she wasn't valuable enough to steal. It was terrible; no matter how hard I tried to explain the circumstances to Carol—*I'm doing this for you*, I whispered—it always made her cry.

◆ ◆ ◆

A Brief Selection of Complaints About a Crying Doll from Amazon:

> We loved the idea that this doll "cried" real tears, however, we realized that when Baby Annabell does cry..her tears pour out soaking everything. Also I was disappointed that her mouth didn't move when crying or laughing. And speaking of crying.....she almost never does![103]

> The tears are a joke also. They do not come at an even flow and are not impressive at all!

> I dont see why all parents have to be so grumpy with this toy. I adore it. The only thing is she only cries out of one eye.[104]

A Complaint About a Crying Doll From Amazon That Could Also Describe Myself Some Days:

> The doll will cry but then nothing else. After it
> cries you hear a mechanical sound inside the doll
> (like it is trying to do something) but nothing
> happens. The sound just keeps grinding until
> you manually turn it off.[105]

+ + +

All the crying baby dolls are white.

+ + +

In 2000, the video artist Tony Oursler created a small rag doll with a blank head onto which he projected a recording of an actor's crying face. Oursler said that his crying doll was "effective" because of its "superhuman ability to never stop weeping, which in turn becomes horrifying for the viewer, who eventually must turn away. It is that moment of turning away which the empathy test is all about."[106] I dislike the term "empathy test," with its suggestion of the artist's own moral superiority, his ability to measure and judge the goodness of others. There's a sneer there beneath the crying, and it is the sneer from which I want to turn, not the tears.

◆ ◆ ◆

It's a trap, a false choice between two bad options: turn away or be held in the helpless position of witnessing suffering you have no power to lessen. I hate this art and its instruction.

◆ ◆ ◆

The bodies of "brain-dead" patients sometimes produce tears when their organs are removed. How strange it is to decide upon a subject for that sentence. I do not feel compelled, for instance, to say that the bodies of footballers sometimes produce tears when they win the World Cup, though that is in its own way true. Other physical stimulation also provokes responses from the brain-dead: they will just barely open their eyes "in response to twisting of a nipple."[107]

◆ ◆ ◆

When Charlotte Perkins Gilman—the woman who proposed the abolition of private kitchens—became pregnant, she fell so ill she could not get out of bed. After giving birth she became even more depressed. In a diary entry typical of its time, in the early years of her daughter's life, she wrote:

> Do not feel well during the day. Sew some on dress. Cold and windy. Good dinner. Get hysterical in the evening while putting K. to sleep. Walter finishes the undertaking, and sleeps with her. When I am nervous she never does sleep easily—what wonder.[108]

+ + +

I do not want to see so much of myself in these lines. I do not want the lives of mothers to have changed so little in 130 years. I am afraid for my daughter's future. I am afraid of coming apart.

+ + +

After college, when I lived in New York, I worked as an assistant for a real estate broker at Prudential Douglas Elliman. I was no good at it—had no context for understanding the social and financial complexities of assembling an application to the board of a wealthy Upper East Side co-op—and my employer's frequent remonstrations often made me cry. One day, at a damp and solitary lunch, I came across a literary map of Manhattan in *The New York Times*, and saw the address of my workplace mid-list. Sylvia Plath had spent an infamous summer there as a young guest editor for *Mademoiselle*, and then wrote about it in *The Bell Jar*. "Well, that's all right, then," I thought, sniffling a little less.

✦ ✦ ✦

But it is dangerous to lay a map of one's own life over another's, to make it a trap. It is dangerous to always think of one thing as another. I wrapped Plath's paragraphs over myself like a winding sheet. In the book, Esther—the protagonist whose experience closely parallels Plath's own—is about to be photographed holding some object meant to represent what she wants to be, but:

> I didn't want my picture taken because I was going to cry. I didn't know why I was going to cry, but I knew that if anybody spoke to me or looked at me too closely the tears would fly out of my eyes and the sobs would fly out of my throat and I'd cry for a week.

> When they asked me what I wanted to be I said I didn't know.

> "Oh, sure you know," the photographer said.

"She wants," said Jay Cee wittily, "to be everything."

I said I wanted to be a poet.

Then they scouted about for something for me to hold.

Jay Cee suggested a book of poems, but the photographer said no, that was too obvious. It should be something that showed what inspired the poems. Finally Jay Cee undipped the single, long-stemmed paper rose from her latest hat.

. . .

"Give us a smile."

At last, obediently, like the mouth of a ventriloquist's dummy, my own mouth started to quirk up.

"Hey," the photographer protested, with sudden foreboding, "you look like you're going to cry."[109]

✦ ✦ ✦

I do not want to cry. I want to be a poet. I want to look at the words with a dry and unswollen face.

• • •

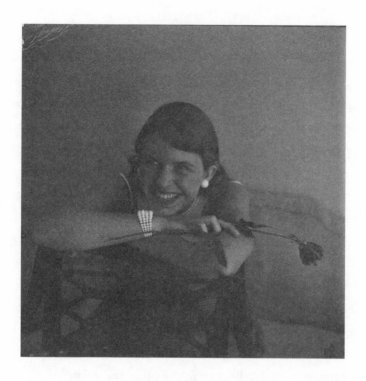

• • •

To *break* into tears seems the right verb, as if one leans on a membrane until it gives way, until the boundary between the body and its tears dissolves, until the citizen self falls into the nation of cry. Or perhaps it is that one's self *becomes* tears, breaks into small, hot droplets. "They cried and cried until they were *all* tears,"[110] says one of the children's board books I've now read a thousand times, and Little Blue and Little Yellow disintegrate on the sturdy page.

⋆ ⋆ ⋆

Last night there was a "black moon," the second new moon in a month. It feels like it wants to be a way of singing, a lunar argument against this country's murderous forces, but it is dangerous to always think one thing is another, every event a metaphor for another, each life and death a reiteration of the ones that came before. "The moon is no door; it is a face in its own right."[111] It is raining, not crying. There is enough grief without trying to wring tears from the moon.

⋆ ⋆ ⋆

Brian Boyd argues that metaphor and story stem in part from humans' tendency to ascribe agency to inanimate objects, that this makes good evolutionary sense, as it is "safer to suppose a bush a bear than the other way around."[112]

⋆ ⋆ ⋆

A few more kinds of moons:

> blood
> super
> harvest
> blue

strawberry

wolf

snow

worm

pink

buck

red

mourning

cold

wet

flower

✦ ✦ ✦

No matter how one orders the moons, story—inchoate—
emerges.

✦ ✦ ✦

In 1944, two psychologists conducted an experiment, showing a brief animated film featuring geometric shapes to a
group of undergraduate women and then asking them to
"write down what happened in the picture." Most descriptions were narrative and patriarchal, despite the shapes' face-
lessness: "A man has planned to meet a girl and the girl comes
along with another man." One resulting answer differed from
all the others in its detached, almost entirely geometrical

description: "A large solid triangle is shown entering a rect-angle ... Then another, smaller triangle and a circle appear on the scene. The circle enters the rectangle while the larger triangle is within." But even this description, by the end, as-signs consciousness, gender, and agency to the shapes: "The larger triangle, now alone, moves about the opening of the rectangle and finally goes through the opening to the inside. He moves rapidly within, and, finding no opening, breaks through the side and disappears."[113]

✦ ✦ ✦

I suppose the least narrative version of the film would be made of ones and zeroes. But even binary code can lead to feelings: on/off, present/absent, yes/no.

✦ ✦ ✦

I have been working so hard not to cry from fatigue and sor-row, and still crying so much, that I've only just realized I cannot recall the last time I wept for some happier or less categorized reason. My sister comes to visit and the sight of her new baby smiling at my daughter brings her to joyful tears. Startled, I stare, recognize the ghost of old feelings. "What do I remember / that was shaped / as this thing is shaped?"[114] What if I could hear among the songs of grief a refrain of sweetness too?

＊ ＊ ＊

Perhaps it would be truest to allow two stories to correspond briefly, to align themselves into one moment as they travel on their separate orbits, to know that the instant of recognition of sameness must not last. Now the moon is a sorrowful face, now "a rock with blue scrapes."[115] The lines are neither parallel nor perpendicular, but two arcs that momentarily intersect before traveling on. A meeting need not be an end.

＊ ＊ ＊

When I am not in despair I can barely even describe it. It is a trap door in my life. A bridge to nowhere. It is only a metaphor, a line. But one I send my love across.

＊ ＊ ＊

It is easy to say "only a metaphor," but the metaphor matters, shapes the way we think. Good is up, bad is down, as George Lakoff and Mark Johnson long ago pointed out in their work on conceptual metaphor.[116] Metaphor is everywhere in science, guiding researchers to new ideas or freezing them in old ones. Even the act of conception itself can be imagined differently if one shifts agency in the metaphor, which the historian Patricia Fara illustrated in a recent panel on women in science: Does sperm barrage an egg until one is aggressive enough to break through and fertilize? Or does an egg regard approaching sperm and elect to pull one in?[117]

+ + +

I've been reading William H. Frey's 1985 book, *Crying: The Mystery of Tears*, a scientific exploration of how and why we cry. Frey led, for several years, experiments on the chemical composition of tears, as well as investigations into crying behavior among adults in the United States. He is a proponent of the idea that crying is an excretory process, that it helps rid the body of stress-related chemicals, and that this may be the reason we feel better after a good cry.[118] (We do not, not always, but you know that already.) When Frey first published his work, the media response was enormous, as viral as it could be in the pre-Internet era. Walter Cronkite interviewed him. Charles Schulz referred to his work in a *Peanuts* cartoon.[119] Curious about that art in particular, I email Frey to ask if he might share it with me, and he soon calls back.

+ + +

In his book, Frey speculates that "higher levels [of the hormone prolactin] may account in part for the fact that women shed tears more often and more readily than men."[120] I can't help noticing that in his conceptual framework men are the default figure, to which women are compared. And he (and every other crying researcher I've read) treats sex as binary and absolute, sex and gender as interchangeable. I go digging and find that differences in prolactin levels emerge in puberty; people categorized by researchers as female experience an increase, those categorized as male a decline. What would happen if Frey were to flip his model, ask why males suffer from a prolactin deficit, and a corresponding inability to cry? Or better still, what if researchers were to treat sex and gender as the varied sets they are? What would the science of tears look like then?

❖ ❖ ❖

"There's so much misinformation out there," Frey tells me. He once saw a woman reading *When Elephants Weep: The Emotional Lives of Animals* on an airplane and asked her what she thought of it. "It's fascinating," she said. "It may be fascinating," he replied, "but it's certainly not accurate."

❖ ❖ ❖

Still, he can be moved. I tell him about finding the hunter's story of killing the crying elephant. "That's awful," he says, and I hear the emotion in his voice, his emotional animal. I tell him about how I cried listening to *The Champ*. He tells me that the best movie he and his team found for eliciting tears was *All Mine to Give*. He became accustomed to hitting

PLAY for his subjects and then running out of the room, so he wouldn't cry himself. He reached the point when even hearing the film's music would bring tears to his eyes. The film's plot—an orphan is charged with finding homes for each of his younger siblings—is based on a true story, and so, the doctor tells me, you can't push the tears away with the comforting thought that it's not real.

◆ ◆ ◆

bell hooks worries that patriarchy cuts men off from feeling, demands they not cry, though age and awareness of mortality may provide a point of re-entry.[121] It's complicated, though. Men can cry about sports, or recollecting bravery in battle. And it changes over time and space—all the weeping of *The Man of Feeling* was viewed with approval by the eighteenth century's cult of sensibility before the Victorians laughed over a later edition's teasing "Index to Tears."[122]

◆ ◆ ◆

When bell hooks describes her own unwelcoming responses to the tears of men she's loved I feel a pang of recognition and guilt. There was a day when Chris wept terribly over spilling water on his laptop, and though I comforted him, I did so with an interior anger and disgust. The crying seemed excessive, irritating, unbecoming. I wanted to shake him the way you are not supposed to shake a baby. And I had proverbs about spilled milk running through my head. It's hard to turn off the allusions. But I knew, even as I felt these things, that they were wrong. He was exhausted; the laptop's demise gave him a hatch to fall through. I had cried my own way through days and weeks and he was living in fear of the moment when I'd fall again into full despair. His university was in a precarious financial state, and talk of cuts and strikes filled his email. He barely had any time to write, to walk, to think freely. I wanted what is tender in me to tend to his signal that he was overcome, in need of help. But it was like that part of my body had fallen asleep.

◆ ◆ ◆

In the Netflix sitcom *Crashing*, which centers around a group of twenty-somethings living in a semi-abandoned hospital in London, one woman discovers she is capable of orgasming during sex only if her fiancé is crying. It makes me think of the Romantic-era erotic interest in lovers' tears mingling together, though her kink seems *highly* dependent on this man crying alone.

◆ ◆ ◆

A poet friend, Eli, tells me that at a certain point in his transition he realized he hardly cried any more. He was happy for the newfound sense of freedom T gave, feeling his "brain lining up with his body for the first time," but the tearlessness was not only a result of that satisfaction.[123] Situations would arise when he'd feel sad, and would expect tears to come as they had before. They did not; they felt "like a sneeze that passes without coming out." Without physical release, the sadness retranslated itself as anger. Now, instead of crying, he practices breathing, finds it a comfort.

◆ ◆ ◆

When Renato Rosaldo's wife and anthropological partner fell to her death during their fieldwork among Ilongot people in the Philippines, he "tried to cry, [he] sobbed, but rage blocked the tears."[124] Of his approach to her body he writes that he "felt like in a nightmare, the whole world around me expanding and contracting, visually and viscerally heaving. Going down I find a group of men, maybe seven or eight, standing still, silent, and I heave and sob, but no tears."[125] It was only in his grief that he began to feel, rather than translate, Ilongot explanations of headhunting. I have no direct words to offer here, but Rosaldo wrote—in the imprecisely general language of anthropology—that "an Ilongot man" would say "rage, born of grief, impels him to kill his fellow human beings. He claims that he needs a place 'to carry his anger.'"[126]

◆ ◆ ◆

Before she died, Michelle Rosaldo wrote of a night when a group of Ilongot friends asked her to play tape recordings they had made years ago of a headhunting ceremony. In the intervening years, headhunting had become impossible, threatened by a combination of conversions to Christianity and a declaration of martial law throughout the land. When the sound of a traditional headhunting song began to play, one man, Tukbaw, left the house. Another, 'Insan, later explained that he had to leave "so that the young boys who had never taken heads would not know of the intensity of his reaction; he had wanted to cry and felt ashamed."[127]

✦ ✦ ✦

I fear the rage of grieving American men, men who—having suffered some loss of one of their narrow sources of self-worth—decide to murder their families along with themselves. I remember walking one day with my sister, who paused to answer a phone call from a friend. She fell in a crumpled crying heap to the sidewalk. News of death. A man who killed his wife—the friend's sister—and then himself. While their children looked on. Unbearable.

✦ ✦ ✦

Judith Butler wonders if it might be possible to find a "[source] of nonviolence in the capacity to grieve, to stay with the unbearable loss without converting it into destruction," or "if the grief is unbearable is there another way to live with it that is not the same as bearing it?"[128]

I wonder whether men kill to create an occasion for the grief they already feel.

❖ ❖ ❖

I learned the other day that water freezes around that which is not water, that it requires a molecule of difference to remember how to form ice, that each snowflake very likely takes shape around a bacterium.[129] An occasion.

❖ ❖ ❖

"Some people don't know how to cry. Some people, when they lose their relatives, they don't know how to talk and cry," says Ami Dokli, a contractor people hire "to go to their funerals and cry for them" in Ghana.[130] Yes, I think, here is the molecule of difference, the one that teaches water to become ice, helps grief remember how to become tears. Dokli offers form, not content, models the shape into which one's mourning might flow.

❖ ❖ ❖

The tears of a professional mourner are like the beats a teacher offers—da DA da DA da DA da DA da DA—to instruct a student in how a body might produce the sound of an iambic foot. But no, Dokli goes on to explain that she and the people she works and weeps alongside are all widows. Their tears are not mere examples of form; they are lines of grief carried over onto a new page.

◆ ◆ ◆

On a snowy morning in 1972, during the presidential primary season, the Democratic candidate Ed Muskie stood outside the *Union Leader* in New Hampshire to defend his wife against the paper's attacks, and reporters wrote that he cried. The story damaged his reputation for strength, and McGovern secured the nomination. Muskie denied that he'd cried, said the tears were only snowflakes that had fallen in his eyes.[131]

◆ ◆ ◆

A 2013 study of "hedonic reversal," or "benign masochism," explores how people find enjoyment in "initially negative experiences that the body (brain) falsely interprets as threatening," such as spicy food, disgusting jokes, or sad music. They posit that the "realization that the body has been fooled, and that there is no real danger, leads to pleasure derived from 'mind over body.' This can also be framed as a type of mastery."[132]

I want to find a way to set mastery aside, so that I seek neither to master that which brings me to tears nor to surrender to it completely. I want neither to master the waves these sentences ride, nor to submit to a buffeting that would only reproduce the harms that already exist. I want to learn to navigate by stars that have nothing to do with me, stars no human can master, but by whose light one might see where to go. I want to point my child toward that light.

+ + +

Butler says,

> Mourning has to do with yielding to an unwanted transformation where neither the full shape nor the full import of that alteration can be known in advance [. . .] Whatever it is, it cannot be willed. It is a kind of undoing. One is hit by waves in the middle of the day, in the midst of a task. And everything stops. One falters, even falls.[133]

+ + +

Bas Jan Ader's words return to me: "When I fell off the roof of my house, or into a canal, it was because gravity made itself master over me. When I cried, it was because of extreme grief."

✦ ✦ ✦

Butler has questions, ones I share:

> What is that wave that suddenly withdraws your gravity and your forward motion? That something that takes hold of you and makes you stop, takes you down?
>
> Where does it come from? Does it have a name?[134]

✦ ✦ ✦

I do not know how to name why I am crying. I mean, I can name some contributing circumstances—sleep deprivation chief among them—but in the moment nothing can adequately explain why my whole consciousness is made of pain. The despair is not reasonable. It has no sense of proportion. It knows the material conditions of my life are not under threat, but it does not care. Collapsed on the floor and in tears, I hear myself tell Chris I am not a real person. I am trying to connect those words to my inability to get up, to wash a plate, to imagine a way to walk to another room, but the gravitational force is so immense that I cannot lift those clauses into speech. The floor is the only thing that can hold me. If I could go any lower I would.

✦ ✦ ✦

Despair makes us fall and a fall makes us laugh. Why? The philosopher Henri Bergson says it is because of the involuntary nature of a fall, that we laugh because "the muscles [continue] to perform the same movement when the circumstances of the case [call] for something else," imagining a man who fell because "[p]erhaps there was a stone in the road. He should have altered his pace or avoided the obstacle."[135]

✦ ✦ ✦

If scientists present images of faces whose tears have been photoshopped away, subjects have difficulty recognizing whether a person is laughing or crying.

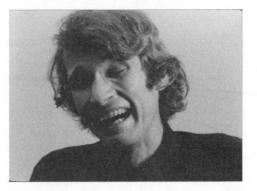

Still from Bas Jan Ader's film *I'm Too Sad to Tell You*

Last week, cutting sweet potatoes for dinner while my daughter played at the sink, I suddenly lost track of my left hand. It was as if, when I moved the hand into a certain location, the location itself vanished. Then everything—all locations, my body, my sense of myself in the world—began to seem unreal, as if there were no me to think, only a kind of narration. *This might*, said the narration, *be a stroke*. I put down the knife. I called a friend. I did this because the narration knew this was how one should act in this story, but I was not afraid. Whatever of me was still there, I have since come to realize, was excited and curious about this new form of consciousness. It was, perhaps, a form of hedonic reversal, only instead of pleasure at the power of the mind over the body, I experienced pleasure at the power of the body over the mind. Or pleasure at the disintegration of the false divide between the two.

✦ ✦ ✦

After a trip to the emergency room and a CT scan, a doctor announces it was not a stroke, only an ocular migraine. I remember a different occasion, years ago, when my vision suddenly went askew, and I was for a short time unable to read words. I'd hold a book up in front of me and see the black symbols, but could not decipher them. They looked to me just as they'd done before I learned how to read: orderly, attractive, incomprehensible. On that day I wept.

＊ ＊ ＊

When I was a child, if my mother wanted to punish me, she'd take away my books. This was after she gave up physical punishment. I remember the last spanking, standing in my bedroom with my hands grasping a shelf, staring hard at my books' colorful spines so as to prevent any tears from falling. I wanted to punish her in return, to make her feel a failure. I turned around to tell her face, *That didn't even hurt.*

＊ ＊ ＊

The day after my daughter was born, the obstetrician who'd cut me open came into my room on his rounds. I wanted to ask him what had made the C-section necessary, what had caused the infection that spurred him toward surgery. I don't remember how I phrased my question, but I can recall with complete precision his reply: "The vagina is a dirty place." The book I would like to have thrown at him? *Our Bodies, Ourselves.* Amazon estimates the shipping weight of the 1973 hardcover edition at 1.3 pounds.

＊ ＊ ＊

At the conclusion of the report on hedonic reversal, the researchers speculate:

Perhaps our most interesting finding is that there is a tendency for some people to enjoy a wide variety of sad experiences and crying at them, and that this tendency is more common in females. More than any other hedonic reversal, the liking for sadness is engaged by works of art; it has an aesthetic quality. If we had a better understanding of the function of sadness, we would no doubt be able to make more sense of this.[136]

✦ ✦ ✦

"If we had a better understanding of the function of gender we would no doubt be able to make more sense of this."

"If we had a better understanding of aesthetics we would no doubt be able to make more sense of this."

"If

"If

"If

"If

◆ ◆ ◆

It is exhausting sometimes to conduct these imaginary arguments with scientists who seem determined to misunderstand the bodies of others. And I fear that even if they were to read these words they would still not take me seriously, that my sad brain and tear-swollen face would discredit me.

◆ ◆ ◆

Some theorists speculate that Margery Kempe's spectacular crying was both genuine ("all tears are real tears," remember) and a performance that gave her religious authority in an age when, as a married woman, she would have had no path to an official position in the church.[137] If one is to access power through tears, however, they must fall according to the codes of the age. Kempe's immense grief before an image of the *pietà*, for instance, shows the depth and truth of her religious experience, and discredits that of the priest who admonishes her, "Woman, Jesus is long since dead."[138] For Kempe all time is one, and Jesus is always dying.

◆ ◆ ◆

When I am lowest, when I am in despair, it feels as if whichever violent death I've learned of most recently is occurring right in front of me, that the suffering has no end to it, that its enormity is matched only by the immensity of my guilt and powerlessness. When I am not in despair I can act. The guilt transforms to responsibility, the powerlessness to resolve.

✦ ✦ ✦

One Sunday I go to a Friends' Meeting. I am not a Quaker, nor do I believe in God, but I am in despair. I go with a copy of Zbigniew Herbert's "Envoy of Mr. Cogito" in my pocket, a talisman upon which to focus in the silence. As soon as I settle into the quiet my body begins to cry. I didn't bring a tissue with me, and have to periodically wipe my dripping nose on my sleeve like a child.

✦ ✦ ✦

In the poem Herbert lists the many natural elements of the world which one must love, and then declares:

> they don't need your warm breath
> they are there to say: no one will console you[139]

✦ ✦ ✦

I keep sharing this poem with people, as it gives me courage—which holds me when I cannot reach hope—but only other poets seem to understand. Other people seem puzzled, concerned. I think they want a poem to be a net, a nest. They want Jesus in a purple robe to console them.

I don't mean to make poets sound special. We are just workers. Always I try to keep this wisdom from Henri Bergson in mind:

> In a play of Labiche there is a character who cannot understand how it is possible to be anything else than a timber merchant. Naturally he is a timber merchant himself. Note that vanity here tends to merge into SOLEMNITY, in proportion to the degree of quackery there is in the profession under consideration. For it is a remarkable fact that the more questionable an art, science or occupation is, the more those who practice it are inclined to regard themselves as invested with a kind of priesthood and to claim that all should bow before its mysteries. Useful professions are clearly meant for the public, but those whose utility is more dubious can only justify their existence by assuming that the public is meant for them: now, this is just the illusion that lies at the root of solemnity.[140]

Writing a poem is not so very different from digging a hole. It is work. You try to learn what you can from other holes and the people who dug before you. The difficulty comes from people who do not dig or spend time in holes thinking that the holes ought not to be so wet, or dark, or full of worms. "Why is your hole not lined with light?" Sir, it is a hole.

✦ ✦ ✦

When Charlotte Perkins Gilman's despair became too great, she wrote to Silas Weir Mitchell, a physician renowned for his "rest cure," a treatment for people (often white women and veterans of war) suffering from "neurasthenia," or a "weakness of the nerves." After spending a month in his care, Gilman returned home with a prescription she recalled years later in her autobiography: "Live as domestic a life as possible. Have your child with you all the time. [. . .] Lie down an hour after each meal. Have but two hours' intellectual life a day. And never touch pen, brush or pencil as long as you live."[141]

✦ ✦ ✦

Some scholars doubt these instructions. They suggest that Gilman's recollection was imperfect, that Mitchell often encouraged women to engage in creative pursuits.[142] I tell you this for the sake of responsibility, pretending to be a scholar myself. In my heart—my sad and irrational heart—I believe her.

✦ ✦ ✦

Gilman's last diary entry before traveling to see Dr. Mitchell:

Tues. April 19th. 1887.

Snowed yesterday. Cold night. Wintry this morning. Another letter from Mrs. Cresson. Take baby to Mary's. Back and lunch. Come over home. Doors locked. No key to be found. Struggle in at bay window with much effort. Clear up and write here. Begin to write an account of myself for the doctor.[143]

* * *

I cannot find any record of that account listed among Mitchell's papers, but I can find his correspondence with Oliver Wendell Holmes, the Autocrat whose words about mentally ill women Mitchell quoted approvingly:

An hysterical girl is, as Wendell Holmes has said in his decisive phrase, a vampire who sucks the blood of the healthy people about her.[144]

* * *

If Mitchell were to find Gilman weeping at the locked door, I imagine he'd think her a pest, a bloodsucking hysteric. I get it. I have stood at that door in tears and thought of myself that way too.

* * *

On Yahoo! Answers people want to know whether or not vampires cry, and—if they do—whether the tears they shed are blood. Responses are inconclusive.

* * *

The most potent tears, I think, are those elicited by some tiny event in the midst of wider tragedy. This is why my heart jumps out to Gilman, keyless, at the door. In the midst of an angry divorce someone runs over a squirrel. The day after the funeral, the laundromat's coin machine won't work. Some people would say that they are not really crying about the coin machine; they are crying about their grief, but like Zach says in that poem:

> the good thing
> about crying is you
> don't really have to
> pick a subject.[145]

* * *

Yesterday my daughter cried because the lemon she wanted to eat did not remain whole. And because she was worried there would not be enough snow.

✦ ✦ ✦

There's that website that catalogs "Reasons My Son Is Crying," and it can be pretty funny: "The goat ate the goat food from his hand,"[146] etc., but I would like it better if it became weirder, more abstract: "The desire to share the object could not be reconciled with the desire to maintain possession of the object." With a photograph for illustration. I think it would make me laugh, not out of joy, but out of surprise at glimpsing the strange grid hovering behind what we can see.

✦ ✦ ✦

Perhaps I am thinking along the lines of Roland Barthes, who wrote in his *Mourning Diary*, after the death of his mother:

> Sad afternoon. Shopping. Purchase (frivolity) of a tea cake at the bakery. Taking care of the customer ahead of me, the girl behind the counter says *Voilà*. The expression I used when I brought *maman* something, when I was taking care of her. Once, toward the end, half-conscious, she repeated, faintly, *Voilà* (*I'm here*, a word we used to each other all our lives).

The word spoken by the girl at the bakery brought tears to my eyes. I kept on crying quite a while back in the silent apartment.

That's how I can grasp my mourning.

[...]

The most painful point at the most abstract moment ...[147]

◆ ◆ ◆

Or else I am thinking of Renee Gladman, who writes of trying to prepare her students to read the poems of Ed Roberson: "Often when reading poetry, it's the grid you're experiencing, and the grid is not the same thing as that subterranean container, where some meaning might lie," though she soon realizes that "there was a flaw to my thinking. The place from which the emanations arose was not intact, it was not a container wherein lay meaning. It was a grid itself but of what I could not explain within the allotted time."[148]

◆ ◆ ◆

The moments when I catch a glimpse of the inexplicable grid feel like the opposite of despair.

Last night I arrived in Philadelphia, ready to spend the week among Mitchell's archive at the Philadelphia College of Physicians' Historical Library. His likeness populates each room, in portrait and bust. His handwriting is nearly indecipherable: the nineteenth-century scrawl of a physician with a hand tremor. Whenever he turns to the typewriter my whole body relaxes.

✦ ✦ ✦

Mitchell's only daughter, Maria, child of his second wife, Mary, became ill with diphtheria just after Christmas 1897. She was twenty-two. By mid-January she was so sick that Mitchell had to tell Mary of "M's perilous state," to which she replied, "I will be quiet. I can endure even this."[149]

✦ ✦ ✦

From Mitchell's diary:

January 22, 1898

My little maid died at 02.30 this accursed day
— we are left alone.

January 24, 1898

Today my child is buried
my wife is ill and
I can not see her
I can bear my grief but have to bear hers

— We left my last maid alone in the hideous
place of graves — & I came back to break up
[to argue] with my Mary when she said she was
lonely —
ah is not all true sorrow lonely — none can share
— so as to make it less —

Then Mitchell, who always longed to be taken more seriously
as a poet, breaks into verse:

There is a grief beyond all other grief
To bear the sorrow of some heart so dear
That this sad burden seems past all relief
That time can bring or faith can give us here
Ye who have suffered what today is mine
are happy if ye escape this added pain
The unbearable anguish that doth [indecipher-
    able]
To weep for those who weep & weep in vain.
God help me.[150]

I knew before I came here that—despite the antagonism I feel toward Mitchell and his disdain for hysterical women—in the intimacy of his letters and diaries I would find some sense of kinship. I did not know I would have to turn my head away so as to avoid damaging the archival materials with tears shed for his grief.

* * *

I pause for lunch and in the break room meet John, a fundraiser for the college who's recently returned from years living abroad. Already primed by my intimacy with Mitchell's papers, I tell John I've just been crying downstairs in the library, and he sweetly shares stories of his own recent tears, the difficulty of coming home. Beth, the librarian, joins us, and I tell her too of my archival weeping. Beth says she cried when she saw the Gutenberg Bible at the British Museum, so profusely that a concerned guard bade her step away.

* * *

Today I met a sexton named Sharon, one of just two people remaining to tend to St. Stephen's Episcopal Church, where the Mitchells erected a memorial to their daughter by the sculptor Augustus Saint-Gaudens. Sharon said the church no longer holds services; the nearby hospital slowly bought up the neighborhood's buildings, and it has virtually no residents left to be parishioners. The grandeur of the church's Tiffany windows argues with the bland, thin carpet. Sharon is a singer as well as a sexton, and she tells me that on Christmas Eve, while singing with a church choir—a setting of a poem by Howard Thurman about "the work of Christmas"—she saw that the choir leader was moved to tears by the song's litany of infinitives. Sharon could not look at the choir leader, because to do so brought tears to her own eyes, and, as she tells me, "You can't sing and cry, you just can't."

◆ ◆ ◆

The pews of St. Stephen's were removed years ago, leaving room for configurations of furniture that change according to the day's needs. As I put on my coat to leave, Sharon begins scooping slimy water from a pool long since abandoned by a visiting meditation group, slowly emptying it into a large bucket. She refuses my offer to help, says she is down to the muck. "Do you sing while you work?" I ask. "Don't tell anyone," she says, "but when I am all alone I come in here to practice."[151]

◆ ◆ ◆

Among the duties of the sexton are the caretaking of the building and its graves. Near the church's entrance lies the recumbent effigy of William Shippen Burd, father to three children buried in a nearby hall beneath a memorial sculpture that shows the children under the gentle eye of the angel of resurrection. The art is too saccharine to elicit my tears, but the people were real, and Sharon is taking care of them when she sings.

◆ ◆ ◆

In 2005, in need of funds and without other options, St. Stephen's sold Maria's memorial to the Philadelphia Art Museum, and it is there I go to gaze upon Saint-Gaudens's work. It does not move me, its smooth marble serenity no match for Mitchell's ragged words. *God help me.*

◆ ◆ ◆

In another wing of the museum, I catch sight of an object whose ingenuity makes me laugh aloud. It's a wooden box. Underneath its lid there's a metal cast of a human foot, and the box itself is full of sand, so that if I were to close it (and I can't, as it's all behind glass), I'd make an artificial footprint. There are even drawers built into the box, so that each footprint can be stored and preserved. "A footprint machine!" I think, and smile. Then I read the placard: Jasper Johns, *Memory Piece (Frank O'Hara)*, and with the smile still on my lips my eyes fill up with tears. I love O'Hara's poems, his enthusiasm, his energy, his exuberant melancholy. He died in 1966 after a dune buggy accident on Fire Island. Johns made the cast of his foot years before O'Hara died, but didn't finish this box until 1970, a bittersweet, faux-naïve act of keeping his friend near, just barely gone, and then—as the sand inevitably settles—vanished.

✦ ✦ ✦

In the folder of an old Hotmail account, I still have dozens of emails from Bill, and sometimes I return to them to see who we were. Once he wrote to tell me he was memorizing "Steps," one of his favorite Frank O'Hara poems, which flits its way through New York, watching dancers in the park:

> who are often mistaken for worker-outers at the
>   West Side Y
> why not
> the Pittsburgh Pirates shout because they won
> and in a sense we're all winning
> we're alive[152]

✦ ✦ ✦

Back at the library, I have spent the morning reading *The Lacrimal System*, laughing sometimes at the dryness with which doctors describe tears. When I see a reference to a 1791 dissertation by two French physicians on the chemical composition of tears it occurs to me that I do not know the French word for crying, and I learn that one could speak of *les pleurs* or *les larmes*. Wanting to find out more about the differences between the terms, I step into Mitchell Hall—an imposing, high-ceilinged meeting room, empty save for grand chairs at the front, the grandest of which Mitchell himself sat in as college president—to text a French-speaking friend. Before I can finish tapping my message, a text arrives from my mother, telling me my godmother has just died, and I feel the eyes of all the presidents—whose portraits people the empty room—fall upon me as my own eyes fill up with tears. The books are correct: psychogenic tearing is always bilateral.

✦ ✦ ✦

I step forward to face Mitchell's chair, which sits beneath his portrait, and try to find a kind of privacy with him, remembering the International Study of Adult Crying's finding that it is best to cry neither alone nor with many others present. One witness will suffice, will give comfort. *Mitchell, are you with me?* It is a long way down for him to look.

✦ ✦ ✦

The Saint-Gaudens sculpture was not the only memorial for Maria. A year after her death, Mitchell privately printed a poem he wrote in her memory, "Ode on a Lycian Tomb," which comments upon a sarcophagus the doctor saw in

Constantinople, on a journey he and Mary took to distance themselves from their grief. Mitchell had sought solace in Tennyson's long poem "In Memoriam," but found it inadequately conveyed the many facets of his own grief. In the sarcophagus he found the art that matched his sorrow, writing to his son:

> The "pleureuses" is not so great but is most affecting—a dozen women in varied attitudes of grief weep all around the marble—you walk around the Sarcophagus and at last are tremendously sorry for these women—these are the finest things here—as far as the Turk goes they are pearls before hogs—[153]

Only he can understand, can interpret. The doctor who held actual tearful women in such suspicious regard looks at weeping stone women abroad and sees they are weeping according to his code and his need. Again my tenderness for him vanishes. His grief grows too smooth and too white.

+ + +

It was an accident that I came across Mitchell's name in the first place, in the acknowledgments section of the first in-depth study of crying. I looked him up because the study's author, Alvin Borgquist, never published again, and it's impossible to track down his papers directly. After finishing the study he seems to have vanished into a private life in Nevada. From the archive of G. Stanley Hall, his college president and editor of the journal where the study first appeared, I learn that Borgquist had trouble making the journey east to Worcester for school,[154] that his former advisor described him disparagingly as a "self-made" type, that he often inadvertently insulted those who were trying to help him.[155] I wonder whether Borgquist cried much himself, homesick for the West, a Mormon working for an atheist.

◆ ◆ ◆

Back home again, I read about the Mexican legend of La Llorona, the ghostly mother who weeps for the children she killed after her husband deserted her,[156] and I can feel a crack open and widen inside my belly. I close the book before it reaches my head.

◆ ◆ ◆

In online, unattributed gatherings of folktales from Ohio, people tell stories of "crying bridges," structures haunted by weeping ghosts, often mothers who drowned themselves and their infants. In one story the women and their children were running away from slave catchers. Is this a retelling of

Margaret Garner's story, like *Beloved*? They've changed it, though. It's not a knife; it's a river.

✦ ✦ ✦

During the election (which is, as Alexander Chee writes, "the election that for now we all speak of only as 'the election,' as if there will never be any other"[157]) some pundits argued that the wall was only a metaphor, a boundary that would be not physical, but made of words, of laws restricting migration. This week new words announced the wall would be real, but still, its reality has to account for miles and miles of rivers, mountains, and other rough terrain which will want to interrupt the physical embodiment of xenophobic rhetoric. Poets online keep reminding one another of Robert Frost's line: "Something there is that doesn't love a wall."[158]

✦ ✦ ✦

So often a metaphor arrives in the physical world with violence. When King Pedro I of Portugal came to the throne he arrested the men who had—years before—murdered his beloved Inês de Castro. Wanting them to suffer the literalization of the anguish he had experienced in grief, Pedro ordered their hearts to be torn out of their bodies, one from the front, the other from the back. There is form here. Pattern. An attempt to intensify the horror by containing it in symmetry.[159]

⁘

A fountain stands where legend has it Inês was killed, and people say the red marks at its base are, in fact, her bloodstains. They call it the Fonte das Lágrimas; in English, "Fountain of Tears."[160]

⁘

From one side of the border the river is called the Rio Grande. From the other it's the Rio Bravo. La Llorona haunts both equally, I imagine. Ghosts are notoriously indifferent to walls.

⁘

When the black veteran speaker of Yusef Komunyakaa's "Facing It" stands looking into the shiny, reflective surface of the Vietnam Veterans Memorial Wall, he wills himself not to cry: "I said I wouldn't, / dammit: No tears. / I'm stone. I'm flesh." The line between the physical and the metaphorical, the wall and the world, blurs, until there seems to be no division between the two:

> A white vet's image floats
> closer to me, then his pale eyes
> look through mine. I'm a window.
> He's lost his right arm

inside the stone. In the black mirror
a woman's trying to erase names:
No, she's brushing a boy's hair.[161]

The white vet's arm is gone, blown off in the war, but the wall somehow contains it, without any promise of return. The wall makes it as invisible as the speaker's dark-skinned face, which fades and hides in the poem's opening lines. The poem is itself a dark, reflective wall.

◆ ◆ ◆

Years ago I heard the poet Lee Ann Roripaugh speak about "Facing It" in a paper on how a poem can function as a therapeutic device which people use to release pain. She described how the neuroscientist V. S. Ramachandran

> created a mirror box, in which mirrors were used in such a way that a mirror reflection of an amputee patient's intact arm was optically superimposed on the felt location of the patient's phantom arm—thereby creating the visual illusion that the phantom arm was now once again resurrected and embodied. When patients were then told to move their intact, existing hands out of the paralyzed, cramped position, while looking at this optical illusion, they not only saw the phantom limb move, but also FELT the

phantom limb move as well. Astonishingly, this seemed to cure the paralysis and pain in some of the phantom limb patients, while in other patients, the phantom limb disappeared altogether, along with the pain.[162]

Roripaugh posits that "Facing It" functions as a kind of mirror box, a place where Komunyakaa—himself a black veteran, like the poem's speaker—can reflect and release the trauma of war. I am always fascinated by work that brings cognitive science and poetry together, and for months afterward I excitedly shared Roripaugh's ideas with anyone who would listen. One day, visiting Clemson University for a literary festival, I chattered on to my host about the paper until she redirected my thoughts. "I wish," said Jillian Weise, "people would stop using phantom limbs as metaphors. It's a reality some of us actually live with."

✦ ✦ ✦

It was Silas Weir Mitchell who first coined the term "phantom limb," during the Civil War, when he witnessed and performed countless amputations on wounded soldiers. He drew upon his observations to write "The Case of George Dedlow," a short story in the voice of a doctor who enlists as a Union soldier, whose arms and legs are amputated, and who suffers from phantom limb pain. (This despite the initial relief Dedlow experiences when surgeons first remove his infected arm: "I have only a recollection that I said, pointing to the arm which lay on the floor: 'There is the pain, and here am I. How queer!'"[163])

❖ ❖ ❖

Mitchell's archive includes surveys of Civil War veterans who report on their phantom limb pain years after. The pain is in no way metaphorical, though the veterans reach sometimes for similes with which to describe it. Some of them report they are more prone to tears than before they were wounded. Mitchell wanted to understand the link between body and mind, wondered how one's sense of self might shift with loss of limb, but I imagine he would have no patience with Weise, who wants to speak for herself and her prosthesis, and who does, vigorously. She critiques Donna Haraway's "A Cyborg Manifesto" as hopelessly "tryborg," with none of the disabled person's actual melding of self and circuitry:

> Haraway is a tryborg: she's not disabled; she has no interface; she uses the term as a metaphor. The strategic move where one group says, "I shall speak for them because they do not exist / do not live here / do not have thoughts" is common of the tryborg. When they are not speaking for us, they may take a detour into animal studies, a field where

they can rest assured that their subjects remain silent.[164]

✦ ✦ ✦

Before the war, before the rest cure, Mitchell spent most of
his time vivisecting snakes.[165]

✦ ✦ ✦

On television, a journalist asks the demagogue if he ever
cries. His reply: "No, I'm not a big crier. I like to get things
done. I'm not a big crier. I'm not someone who goes around
crying a lot. But I know people like that. I know plenty of
people that cry. They're very good people. But I have not
been a big crier."[166]

✦ ✦ ✦

Byzantine physicians wrote that you could recognize a were-
wolf by its tearlessness.[167]

✦ ✦ ✦

Next month I will fly to Albany on my way to give a reading
in Vermont. Zach will fly there too, will also give a reading.
It has been six years since Bill was buried. It has been twelve

years since Zach published Bill and me in the "new poets" issue of *Octopus*. Now I am what they call a "mid-career" poet and Bill is a dead one.

+ + +

And I am angry with Ted Berrigan, because Bill loved him and Berrigan taught him how to die young. And I am angry with Deborah, because she taught me the poems of these death-facing women and I understood them to be my mothers. And I am angry because the last time I saw her—at a gym, of all places, where I was a receptionist and she was a member—she called me *kiddo* and it was so tender that the word has never left me; I use it to call my daughter, and I do not want to teach her this pattern, this line.

+ + +

Once, after the abortion, Bill wrote to me, "you will have a baby and you will love the baby and the baby will love you and then you will have another baby and that baby will love you and you will have lots of toys and games and love."[168] So far, one baby in, he is right.

+ + +

I wish I could love him again, and better.

Some nights—many nights—Chris and I wake to the sound of our child wailing. We rush to her room to help her, but she is not actually awake. She is having a night terror, stuck at the border between sleep cycles, conscious enough to sense that something is terribly wrong, but not enough to recognize our presence. If I touch her, I am a monster; her crying grows louder, more frantic. All we can do is stand guard, keep her safe.

＊　＊　＊

If I had a prayer, it would say, *Let this not be a mirror to the past, nor a window to the future. Let each night be only itself. Let my child's life find its own peace.*

＊　＊　＊

After I lived in New York, before I moved to Massachusetts for grad school, I spent a summer house-sitting in New Hampshire. Bill and I kept writing to each other. I told him of my nights waiting tables, of my uncle's struggle with leukemia. He replied with his customary lack of capitalization:

> i have been losing friends and making new
> friends. where are you? i keep budging music

folk to let me write songs for them. i'd be good at that. i won't play offense against you. maybe defense. i'll probaly never not want to talk to you. i'm falling for a girl that is in a heavy metal band. i have to stop that. i should move to montreal. open a bar or a bookstore and help stray dogs and write collaged manic poems. i'm half way there. my sentances are jabby. i should come to new hampshire, but i don't know how i'll find time. hopefully. canoes kind of scare me though. the effort that is involved in rowing. sorry about your uncle. i hope you're doing ok. i've been thinking about my father a lot. memories. some of them i think i've completly made up.[169]

✦ ✦ ✦

Bill's father died when he was young too. It was a pattern Bill saw as fate. A line. A look. A family resemblance.

✦ ✦ ✦

My mother comes to visit and we go out to a café to build a timeline of her and our family history, writing each event on a small blue Post-it note. *Nannie and Grandad move to Kew. Mom's house fire. Nannie and Grandad move to Hatch*

End. Mom moves to the kibbutz. If we write it down I can understand.

◆ ◆ ◆

When my English grandparents' marriage was on the verge of falling apart they decided to start over, moving to South Africa, where my aunt was already living with her husband and young children. My mother, whose flat had recently been destroyed in a fire, went with them. She was twenty years old. On the ship she met a white South African, and upon arrival went to stay with him in Johannesburg. My grandparents stayed with my aunt in Pretoria, until my grandfather went to go start a job in Cape Town. After a month he sent word to his family that he was moving back to England, leaving my grandmother.

◆ ◆ ◆

When my grandmother learned of her husband's departure she became suicidal. This is not how she would put it. This is not how my family would put it. Instead, "she could not be trusted with pills." I do not know how her state of mind shifted, but after a time she returned to England—as did my mother—and my grandparents reconciled.

This all happened in 1966, the year Dimitri Tsafendas assassinated Hendrik Verwoerd, the "architect of Apartheid."[170] Verwoerd was largely responsible for laws that forced black South Africans to live in government-designated "homelands," and which forbade black students from attending "white universities." Before his career as a politician, Verwoerd had worked as a psychologist. In 1926 he published an article, "A Method for the Experimental Production of Emotions." His method did not produce tears, but it did produce *satisfaction, disappointment, compassion, regret, exaltation, delight, fear, relief, shame, embarrassment, relief, malicious joy, anger* (and *vexation*).[171] Tsafendas—a multiracial, schizophrenic man who was not allowed to live with his girlfriend because of the country's bewilderingly complicated system of racist classifications—stabbed Verwoerd in the throat and chest. Tsafendas is buried in an unmarked grave in Krugersdorp. Verwoerd is buried in Pretoria, in the "Heroes' Acre."

+ + +

That Christmas my mother's breakdown began. By January she was a patient at Banstead Hospital, which had dropped "Mental" from its name in 1937.[172] She does not remember who drove her there, but she remembers therapeutic art activities, working with tiles and paint. In the room where patients recovered from electroshock therapy she remembers a table with puzzles on it. *There were chairs where I'd sit,* she tells me, *and suddenly realize I was there.*

◆ ◆ ◆

She tells me at first she was not among the electroshock patients, that she watched smugly as those who would receive treatment that day began their morning with no breakfast, while her own tray steamed before her. And then one day, no tray.

◆ ◆ ◆

Later I reread *The Bell Jar* and find Plath's protagonist, Esther, going through the same humbling process:

> At Caplan a lot of the women had shock treatments. I could tell which ones they were, because they didn't get their breakfast trays with the rest of us. They had their shock treatments while we breakfasted in our rooms, and then they came into the lounge, quiet and extinguished, led like children by the nurses, and ate their breakfasts there.[173]

And then one day, for Esther, no tray.

* * *

I wonder whether my mother's memory is made halfway of a book.

* * *

In Verwoerd's experimental method for producing emotions, some participants were asked to punish their partners for making mistakes in a color-recognition game. The punishment was a mild but unpleasant electric shock.[174]

* * *

My mother remembers walking the grounds, the walls of which still stand, though the hospital has since been converted to a women's prison. It keeps shifting back and forth between these two purposes. In the '40s the government requisitioned the building to house prisoners of war.

* * *

I ask my mother what else she remembers of the building, of its corridors and rooms. But it was so long ago. I think of Bachelard's *Poetics of Space*, how he quotes Rilke remembering a building from childhood:

I never saw this strange dwelling again. Indeed, as I see it now, the way it appeared in my child's eye, it is not a building, but is quite dissolved and distributed inside me: here one room: there another, and here a bit of corridor which, however, does not connect the two rooms, but is conserved in me in fragmentary form. Thus the whole thing is scattered about inside me, the rooms, the stairs that descended with ceremonious slowness, others, narrow cages that mounted in a spiral movement, in the darkness of which we advanced like the blood in our veins.[175]

❖ ❖ ❖

What fragments of her history live in my body? What rooms does my blood remember?

❖ ❖ ❖

It's possible that the higher protein content in emotional tears evolved because it increases their viscosity, slows the rate at which they fall, increasing the chance they will be seen and their message received. My mother's tears are watery and streaming now. I wonder if this thinness comes with age. I am watching the tears course along her wrinkles, and I love her face. I am imagining the suffering I would feel if I were speaking this way to my daughter.

I am imagining the youth my mother was, the tears she shed alone.

"I'm sorry," she says, and tries to smile at me. I reach across the salt and pepper on the table and tell her it's okay.

◆ ◆ ◆

When I was a child, *Return to Oz*—the unofficial sequel to the first movie I loved—terrified me. Dorothy is back in Kansas and she can't sleep. Nobody believes her stories. Aunt Em brings her to a frighteningly calm doctor, who plans to treat the child with electrotherapy. Dorothy's acquiescence is not consent.

"Will it hurt?" she asks.

"No no. No no no. It just manages an electrical current," replies the doctor, speaking half to Dorothy, half to her aunt. "The brain itself is an electrical machine. It's nothing but a machine."

Later, when Dorothy's treatment is about to begin, the doctor peers down at her on the gurney.

"Hello Dorothy, how are you?"

"I wish I wasn't tied down."

I wonder what it was like for my mother to watch me watch this film again and again. For her, electrotherapy was an act of care, an intervention that helped her come through the breakdown and back into her life. On the other side of the treatment there was work, and making art. There was marriage to a sailor, and two children in rapid succession. There was emigration, a new country. There was a green card and several wars and the night she would hear me sing my own wish to destroy myself. No, that was still in the future. I wonder if she wanted to tell me any of this while Dorothy quaked on the gurney, lightning filling the window.

* * *

While we're driving to the airport I tell my mother that I'm grateful for the way we spoke, for the openness between us. I tell her I am less afraid now of her death. She tells me about the last time she saw her own mother. She asked Nannie if everything was all right between them. My mind fills with all the things that could have still been wrong, with all the suffering my mother endured, but her mind moves differently. "Yes," her mother told her, "everything is wonderful." And I believe her. I believe her enough.

"And us?" my mother asks. "Is everything all right between us?" I can hear her voice changing, the roughness of encroaching tears.

"Yes," I say, and I take my hand from the wheel to place it over hers. "Everything is wonderful." And I mean it. I mean it enough.

◆ ◆ ◆

This morning everyone is sharing the BBC video of Mathias delivering his dreams to subscribers, riding his bicycle from house to house, and talking about finding a way to put his writing at the center of his life. He looks happy. His yellow pants look happy. His head looks safe inside its helmet.

◆ ◆ ◆

I'm chopping onions for dinner when a professor on a podcast describes a medieval statue of the Virgin Mary whose miraculous tears were, in fact, generated by the movements of fish swimming around in a chamber of water hidden inside her head. The chamber was filled nearly to the brim, so that if a few fish had a moment of simultaneous vigor, the water would slosh about and spill from holes in Mary's eyes.[176] Or that is the story. I can find no other reference to the statue's existence. Another scholar speculates it could be a bit of Reformation-era anti-Catholic propaganda.[177] I don't care; I'm in love with the fish. Of all the lives a fish could lead, imagine it being this one.

+ + +

When I think of this statue it feels like I have moved into that dream Mathias wrote for my child when she was newborn, of watching in the mirror a baby who is not herself. I am remembering: *Inside its mouth there is a fishbowl & some fishes are swimming around in circles. This makes you laugh. You know that when you grow up you will be filled with fishes & they will make you happy & strong.* I would like to grow this way. I would like to find myself full of these wondrous fish, crying and laughing and strange.

+ + +

Zach and I meet up at the car rental kiosk in the Albany airport. We are on our way to give readings at Bennington College, but first we drive to the cemetery where Bill and the posthumously slandered Sara Weed are buried. It is raining, like in a movie. I brought two umbrellas. Zach picks the blue one. Mine is black and white. We follow the map to the section where Weed is buried. I know, from the photos, to look for a tall pedestal with a weeping woman on top. Our steps are loud in the wet late-winter grass. "Look," I say. "There she is." She is so small. I say it to Zach. "She is so small."

♦   ♦   ♦

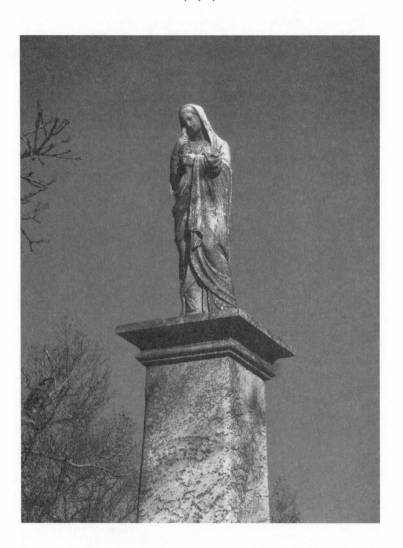

✦ ✦ ✦

We get back in the car and drive to get closer to Bill. The cemetery is enormous, a whole city unto itself. Grand mausoleum mansions, little grave shacks. We drive as far as we can, and then walk up a long hill, following a highlighted blue line along a map the caretaker sent me. It reminds me of the artist Francis Alÿs, who in 1995 walked out of a gallery in São Paolo carrying a dribbling can of blue paint, letting a line leak behind him as he walked through the city, eventually returning to his starting point.[178]

✦ ✦ ✦

I am glad Zach is there. I recite the night of bleeding, how Bill held me through it. I tell him of the growing distance, of Bill's scorn and skepticism when anything went well. "It was easier," I say, and realize as I am saying it, "for Bill to trust me when I was suffering." Another room in my brain recites Dickinson: "I like a look of Agony / because I know it's true."[179] I am suddenly angry with her. With Bill. With myself. Enough. Enough.

✦ ✦ ✦

It is hard to find him. The map is very wet. And then he is there, a rectangle, engraved flat on the ground. His father is buried beside him. I kneel and my knees are wet. I can't speak anything aloud. In my head I am sorry. In my head I read him "Steps." Zach is, I think, just behind me, but the umbrella obscures my peripheral vision. I have forgotten tissues again and wipe my nose on my sleeve.

◆ ◆ ◆

When researchers work to determine whether crying behavior is present, they check against a list, including *touching the eye area, hiding the face, mouth control,* and *gazing up.* Hans Znoj, a psychologist, created the list by asking subjects to remember and speak to a dead spouse as if they were present in the room, and then observing all that happened around the resulting tears. The crying expert Ad Vingerhoets elaborates that "*Gazing up* is effortful and often very brief," which "might be a sign of 'fighting' tears, or it could occur [because] the bereaved person was instructed to talk to the deceased individual, who might be imagined as located in a higher place than the study participant."[180]

◆ ◆ ◆

Bill is not up. The umbrella is up, and black and white, and Bill is beneath my wet knees.

◆ ◆ ◆

Walking back down the hill we talk of suicide, of what it is to lose someone to it, or to fear that loss. I find myself telling Zach

I have felt close to it myself, but I do not want to scare him, so I tell him I am okay now. And I think for now it is true.

◆ ◆ ◆

Bill thought I would be okay. And he thought that he would die. Before thirty, he said. And his prediction was true but that does not mean it was right. It did not—does not—have to be this way, I think. I am still trying to argue with him, to break the parallel line.

◆ ◆ ◆

When we get back in the car I plug in my phone to charge, and the car stereo somehow extracts from it—at random—a song. Joy Division: "Love Will Tear Us Apart." These are the words inscribed on the grave of the lead singer, Ian Curtis. He killed himself when he was twenty-three.

◆ ◆ ◆

The next song—again, random—is the Smiths' "Cemetry Gates." Is this really happening? It is like living inside a book. When, after a while, Zach needs to charge his phone, and the car starts to play a song by St. Thomas—a Norwegian singer whose death was attributed to "not a suicide, but an unfortunate combination of prescribed drugs"[181]—we decide the book is becoming unkind. I turn the stereo off.

* * *

I say book. I mean poem. I mean the way the landscape suddenly reveals itself in layers, a vertical light shining its connective beam from one moment to the next. An entry into—an awareness of—a dimension always present. Not always seen. I think if I can keep myself alive to it, it will keep me from going under.

* * *

The next day Zach and I are nervous because we learn that Mary Ruefle, whose books we both adore, will be coming to our reading. And then she is so kind. She comes to dinner and we go outside for a smoke. She shows us the moon, the extraordinary moon, a dark gray circle with a bright crescent cradling it from below. "The old moon in the new moon's arms," she quotes, and tenderness courses through me.

* * *

It was looking back at Earth that made Alan Shepard cry on the moon. Home. Where he came from.

* * *

After dinner Mary tells us that one way to preserve tears is to let them fall onto black construction paper, that the salt crystals form white splotches on the page. Stars in the night.

◆ ◆ ◆

The history of the lachrymatory—the vial for saving tears—is an imaginary one. Stories of people weeping into tear bottles are probably stories, not records of acts. *The Romans used to do it*, exclaim the Victorians. *The Victorians used to do it*, exclaim sellers on Etsy.[182] Apparently it doesn't work in practice; we don't shed tears copiously enough, and they evaporate too quickly.

◆ ◆ ◆

In a poem, in a dream, we can make as many tears as needed, can follow, like Dara does, a river until we find its source, a bull at a drive-in movie:

> Whatever it is
> on the movie screen
>
> is such that
> it is causing this bull to weep.
>
> He is weeping buckets.
> He can't stop crying.

His tears stream down
his big bull cheeks.

And it is his crying
that's filling up the river.[183]

+ + +

At a university, students have calculated that it is not possible for every human on Earth to cry enough in a day to fill even the world's shortest river. We could, however, fill an Olympic swimming pool, if each of us committed to shedding fifty-five tears.[184]

+ + +

The scientists are not always so kind in their imagining and curiosity. There is an image I cannot loosen from my mind, a fuzzy black circle with a few white geometrical shapes, produced by the researcher Willy Kühne in 1876:

> An albino rabbit was fastened with its head facing a barred window. From this position the rabbit could see only a gray and clouded sky. The animal's head was covered for several minutes with a cloth to adapt its eyes to the dark, that is to let rhodopsin accumulate in its rods. Then

the animal was exposed for three minutes to the light. It was immediately decapitated, the eye removed and cut open along the equator, and the rear half of the eyeball containing the retina laid in a solution of alum for fixation. The next day Kühne saw, printed upon the retina in bleached and unaltered rhodopsin, a picture of the window with the clear pattern of its bars.[185]

+ + +

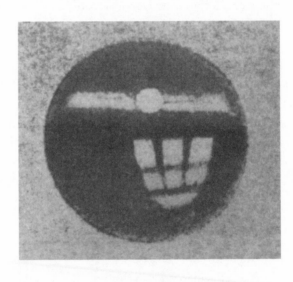

+ + +

In the years that followed the publication of Kühne's study, the idea took hold in the popular imagination that the retinas of a recently deceased person would always show the last image they saw before their death. Police sometimes took pictures of a murder victim's retinas in the hopes of discovering the identity of the killer. Kühne—despite his professed skepticism for this kind of forensic work—himself performed a grotesque investigation of the retinas of a man executed for the murder of his children. He found the results unsatisfactory.[186]

◆ ◆ ◆

I fear that, were someone to examine my retinas after my death, they would find an image of my own hand. "See— here it is— / I hold it toward you."[187]

◆ ◆ ◆

If I had a prayer, it would say, *Let my hands find some other work. Let my hands find my husband's, my child's. A pen, a garden, a phone.*

◆ ◆ ◆

Gabrielle is leading a "somatic workshop on embodying justice," and so I am slowly walking around a gymnasium with a group of twenty other people, arms lifted. We are imagining that each of us is carrying justice. The electricity has gone out all over town, and so the gym—which would normally be filled with the noise of cooling, the buzz of fluorescent lights—is quiet and dim. In the quiet of the work tears come to me and I am ashamed. I try to carry justice to the edges of the room, where my tears won't do something stupid or hurtful. Gabrielle instructs us to find a partner, and for pairs to gaze at each other in silence. I do not know this person, and I am afraid of crying more. Gabrielle says that if laughter comes we should allow it, but she does not mention tears. Later we try to carry justice with our eyes closed, a partner guarding and guiding us. One woman carries justice right out the door. This causes joy and excitement among us. How quickly we accepted the walls of the gym as the limits of the world. How she broke beyond them.

◆ ◆ ◆

I do not mean to make her into some kind of magical figure. She didn't levitate out of that room. She just walked. Outside, to where there was light.

◆ ◆ ◆

Gabrielle looks at *les pleurs* and sees—hears—a softness, the rhyme of fleurs, *flowers*. She looks at *les larmes* and sees war, the hardness of *arms*. Migiwa says that in Japanese, a minuscule amount of something is called "a sparrow's tear."[188] Another friend tells me that in Spanish, *llanto retenido* refers to holding tears in so tightly that you burst "like a volcano," if someone tries to comfort you with touch.[189]

* * *

Or maybe an eruption is too strong an image. Maybe it is more like the tears have filled a vial and formed at the top a meniscus, a curve of surface tension rising above the vial's edge, impossibly full, yet held together by the force of the molecules' attraction to one another. A person touches you, the gentlest touch, they brush a strand of hair from your face, or even just utter words you would call *touching*, and the meniscus, disrupted, falls apart. A fluid slowly leaks over the sides.

* * *

It is story time at the library and I am in a rage. The librarian has taught the children a song:

> May there always be sunshine
> May there always be blue skies
> May there always be Mama
> May there always be me[190]

First the song makes me cry with its plain and painful refusal to acknowledge the impossibility of its wishes. I can tell the song is hurting me because I feel it die in my throat, hear my voice break. *You can't sing and cry, you just can't.* And then the librarian invites the children to shout out their own additions, their own ideas of the things they most love, most want to exist forever. If a child contributes a word that conforms to the librarian's narrow vision of young imagination, she laughs and adds it to the song: "May there always be ice cream / May there always be Grandma." When a child contributes a word outside those irritating limits—carrots, Frodo—the librarian makes an exaggerated taken-aback face, says, "Well I haven't heard *that* before," and adds the word to the song with a look of "What can you do?" It feels as if I can watch the spark of the strange, the spark of the limitless, flicker and struggle under her dampening force. I am so angry.

❖ ❖ ❖

If you cry too much, too hard, it can become its own trauma, can physically alter your throat. An article published in the *Journal of Voice* in 2000 recounts the experiences of three professional singers whose voices became hoarse following heavy crying episodes. A thirty-four-year-old mezzo-soprano cried from homesickness. A twenty-six-year-old music teacher experienced "extensive crying while on the phone with her boyfriend." A twenty-seven-year-old soprano sobbed because she had to leave her job and family to sing in a new city. If this were a fairy tale, one singer would learn to moderate her tears, or would decide to return home. She would be rewarded with jewels or marriage. But this is a scientific gathering of case studies. All were diagnosed with "vocal fold hemorrhage," and did not recover fully until the crying-induced injuries were microsurgically repaired.[191]

+ + +

We have driven to visit my family in New Hampshire. The house's small rooms, whose proportions have not shifted much since they were built in 1812, are filled, not just with people—my mother, my father, my sister, her toddler, Chris, our child, myself—but our moods. These are unnamed, but vibrating at such a high frequency it seems like they might develop bodies of their own.

+ + +

Today it is my turn to go into another room to cry. I lie down on the sofa bed and try to locate equilibrium. My eye looks to the right and I realize that this is the window I broke with my head when I was fourteen. Which pane? The invisible one. It lacks the pretty, distorting swirls of the house's original glass. I can look right through it to the other side.

+ + +

I go to the brewery because I need to write a blurb and my blurbs come out better if I write them in public. The book, by Kate Colby, is tremendous, and begins with an epigraph from Kate Greenstreet that could serve as an epigraph for any book, or life, or world: "Things go together because they are together." David Bowie is playing on the speakers and there is some strange and wonderful person wearing beige pants and a matching beige visor and it all goes together so beautifully that I cry.

◆　◆　◆

At lunch with Gabrielle I try to describe the feeling of this, the joy of being among ideas without writing them down. As when driving a car toward lunch with a friend. At such moments, I say, I am *dispersed with thought.* I have the sense that my consciousness begins in and then extends beyond my body, like dust motes riding alongside me, catching the light.

◆　◆　◆

But there is delight, too, in shaping words around the thoughts. I like it. People like it. People like Anne Carson, who—having already shaped words around falling—goes on to say:

> My favorite part is connecting the ideas. The best connections are the ones that draw attention to their own frailty so that at first you think: *what a poor lecture this is—the ideas go all over the place* and then later you think: *but still*

what a terrifically perilous activity it is, this activity of linking together all the threads of human sin that go into making what we call sense, what we call reasoning, an argument, a conversation. How light, how loose, how unprepared and unpreparable is the web of connections between any thought and any thought.[192]

◆ ◆ ◆

I have been afraid I would die while writing this book. I have been afraid all the connections are wrong. And I also have not known how to stop. The crying does not stop; the web could grow forever. So how does one end?

◆ ◆ ◆

One day, Harriet—my child, the child who has grown into her name while years grew around this work—she finds the handwritten draft of a bad poem lying on the table next to a highlighter.

"What's this, Mama?"

"It's a highlighter."

"What's it for?"

"You use it to color in the words you like."

And—though her literacy extends only to knowing the alphabet, not yet to independently deciphering full words—she picks up the highlighter and carefully selects the words to which her eye feels drawn. When she walks off I pick up the poem, which her revisions have immeasurably improved:

> where you have not
> remembered to be sad
> suddenly
> not sung
>
> small knife
>
> that is
>
> I live
> long enough
> there

✦ ✦ ✦

In Wonderland when Alice nearly drowns in her own tears she seeks help from a nearby paddler: "O Mouse, do you know the way out of this pool? I am very tired of swimming about here, O Mouse!"[193]

✦ ✦ ✦

I have cried every day this week, at times for hours. I hear myself describe the intensity of the tears, myself sobbing on the kitchen floor for no reason, "like a madwoman." Why "like"? In these moments I am one. I am. An equation that can be simplified to this point—x = x—is called an *identity*.

✦ ✦ ✦

But there is another way to say it. An identity is also an equation that is true regardless of which real number one substitutes for *x*. "Rose is a rose is a rose is a rose."[194]

✦ ✦ ✦

When Stein says it that way the identity refracts, casts new light. Yes, I want that. My beloved Alexander Vvedensky did too, wanted to discover "unknown real relations" between things. How?

> I doubted that, for instance, house, cottage, and tower come together under the concept of building. Perhaps the shoulder must be linked to the number four. I did it practically, in my poems, as a kind of proof. And I convinced myself that the old relations are false, but I don't

know what the new ones must be like. I don't even know whether they should form one system or many.[195]

◆ ◆ ◆

I do not know either. But I know I need to stop crying for long enough that I regain my capacity to imagine possibilities again.

◆ ◆ ◆

I pause my crying to go give a craft talk at a nearby university. It is about the impossible, about how art—and poetry in particular—can make the limits of our imagining apparent at the very moment it moves beyond them. For just a moment. I tell the story of the woman walking out of the gym. We watch a clip of *Duck Soup*, see a real dog emerge from Harpo Marx's doghouse tattoo, laugh at its impossible bark. We marvel at how Danez Smith reconfigures the possibilities of the physical world through joyfully reimagined positions for sex: "Reverse-Reverse Cowgirl aka Someone get / that horse off that woman! We kill the horse. / We ride its ghost into the sunset."[196]

When I ask if someone would be willing to read Aram Saroyan's one-word poem "lighght"[197] aloud, a poet says, "I will," walks to the corner of the room, and switches the lights rapidly on and off.[198]

We all flicker. For just a moment, we have moved inside the poem.

If you are struggling with thoughts of self-harm or suicide, there are people you can talk to. Call the National Suicide Prevention Lifeline at 1-800-273-8255 for help in the United States. In Canada, call 1-833-456-4566.

Acknowledgments

When a book comes into being over so many years, one's debt to others grows very large. I have needed much from—and been given much by—people whose generosity and grace astonishes me. My gratitude to all of you:

Those whose writing, art, and other creations consoled, stimulated, and instructed me, whose names appear throughout these pages.

Those who gave me shelter and sustenance while I worked away from home: Molly Brodak, Blake Butler, and Dara Wier.

Those who read drafts of the manuscript, offered their critiques, held me accountable, and buoyed me onward in the work: Kaveh Akbar, Nuar Alsadir, Michele Christle, Gabrielle Civil, Madeline ffitch, Rachel B. Glaser, Paige Lewis, Lisa Olstein, and Emily Pettit.

Those who corresponded or conversed with me about particular passages in the book and its surrounding texts, for the gifts of their time, attention, expertise, and care: Erik Ader, Kim Albrecht, Benjamin Bearnot, Roger Beebe, Joan Blackburn, Misha Botting, Dorothée Bouquet, Gillian Brown, Bogdana Carpenter, Meghan Cassidy, Nancy Cervetti, Yi-Fei Chen, Julia Cohen, Megan Cook, John Crawford Jr., Sharon Derstine, Matt Ellis, Charles Fairbanks, Jessica Fjeld, William H. Frey, Ross Gay, Steve Henn, Ilya Kaminsky, Danielle Litwak, Migiwa Orimo, Eugene Ostashevsky, Bomani Moyenda, Eli Renaud, Karen Rommelfanger, Sammy Saber, Zachary Schomburg, Michael and Judy Schurer, Christina Sharpe, Jessica Smith, Jordan Stempleman, Mathias Svalina, Moriel Rothman-Zecher, Jeanette Van Der Breggen, Eleanor Villforth, Lewis Wallace, Jillian Weise, and Betsy Wheeler. In particular, I'd like to thank Natalie Lyalin, who devoted many hours to assisting with translation of permission requests.

Those whose work in libraries and archives made ideas, words, and images accessible: Beth Lander at the Historical Medical Library at the College of Physicians in Philadelphia; Christeene Alcosiba, Rhonda Wynter, and Kathy

Shoemaker at the Stuart A. Rose Library at Emory University; Fordyce Williams at Clark University's Archives and Special Collections; Karen Kukil at Smith College's Young Library; Sarah McElroy Mitchell and Penny Ramon at Indiana University's Lilly Library; Declan Smith at the BBC; Morgan Swan at Dartmouth College's Rauner Special Collections Library; and Elisabeth Stürmer at the Munich Stadtmuseum.

Those whose financial support made research-related travel and other work possible: the Francis Clark Wood Institute for the History of Medicine of the College of Physicians of Philadelphia, the Rose Library Short Term Fellowship Program at Emory University, and the Ohio Arts Council.

Those whose work brought this book into the world: Leigh Newman, my editor at Catapult, whose careful reading of the page's strands made new patterns possible; Sarah Castleton, my editor at Corsair; Annika Domainko, my editor at Hanser; Sabine Huebner, my German translator, whose thoughtful questions illuminated all I hoped these words might do; and my agent, Meredith Kaffel Simonoff, who—from our very first conversation—proved herself a perfect reader for the book, a vital collaborator in its growth, and a trustworthy navigator of its path into publication.

Those whose expert and tender care for my child made space in which I could write: Bert Struewing, Cassandra Powers,

Stephanie Sullivan McClean, and Melanie and Edward Ricart.

Those whose familial love and care have made my life and work possible: my sister, my mother, and my father.

My husband, Christopher DeWeese, who has loved and supported every part of me through every part of our life together.

And our beloved child, whose precious life and story will be her own.

Notes

1. Ovid, "The Art of Love," in *The Art of Love*, trans. Rolfe Humphries (Bloomington: Indiana University Press, 1957), 162.
2. Lauren M. Bylsma, Ad J. J. M. Vingerhoets, and Jonathan Rottenberg, "When Is Crying Cathartic? An International Study," *Journal of Social & Clinical Psychology* 27, no. 10 (December 2008): 1179, Psychology and Behavioral Sciences Collection, EBSCOhost (accessed September 26, 2017).
3. Michael Trimble, *Why Humans Like to Cry: Tragedy, Evolution, and the Brain* (Oxford: Oxford University Press, 2012), 44.
4. Ibid., 37.
5. In an early draft of this book I wrote that "almost nobody cries about sculpture," but then Betsy Wheeler shared with me an image of the Degas sculpture—*Little Dancer*—that brought her to tears. I shifted the sentence to "almost nobody cries about architecture," but then Nuar Alsadir told me about reading of a Sufi building designed in such a way that anyone would begin crying within forty-five seconds of entering. I have since come to

understand that the phrase "almost nobody" has an agenda with which I disagree.

6. W. Derham, "A Short Dissertation Concerning the Child's Crying in the Womb. By the Reverend Mr. W. Derham, F.R.S.," *Philosophical Transactions* 26 (January 1708): 488, doi:10.1098/rstl.1708.0076.

7. W. Derham, "Part of a Letter from the Reverend Mr. W. Derham, F.R.S., to Dr. Hans Sloane, R.S. Sec., Giving an Account of a Child's Crying in the Womb," *Philosophical Transactions* 26 (January 1708): 485, doi:10.1098/rstl.1708.0075.

8. "Elyse (Scott) Green Oral History," Kent State University Libraries, Special Collections and Archives, accessed September 26, 2017, omeka.library.kent.edu/special-collections/items/show/1638.

9. Alice Morby, "Eindhoven Graduate Designs a Gun for Firing Her Tears," *Dezeen Magazine*, November 2, 2016, www.dezeen.com/2016/11/02/tear-gun-yi-fei-chen-design-academy-eindhoven-dutch-design-week-2016. For more on Yi-Fei Chen's project, see neural.it/2017/07/tear-gun-fragility-loaded-weapon.

10. Ad Vingerhoets, *Why Only Humans Weep: Unraveling the Mysteries of Tears* (Oxford: Oxford University Press, 2013), 147.

11. Joe Wenderoth, "January 1, 1997 (New Year's Day)," in *Letters to Wendy's* (Amherst, Mass.: Verse Press, 2000), 142.

12. Chelsey Minnis, "'A woman is cry-hustling a man & it is very fun,'" in *Poemland* (Seattle/New York: Wave Books, 2009), 85.

13. Ross Gay, "Weeping," in *Catalog of Unabashed Gratitude* (Pittsburgh: University of Pittsburgh Press, 2015), 42.

14. "The Sinking of the USS *Indianapolis*," *Witness*, BBC Radio; WYSO, Yellow Springs, Ohio, July 28, 2013.

15. James Matthew Barrie, *Peter Pan: A Fantasy in Five Acts* (New York: Samuel French, 1956), 21.

16. Fanny D. Bergen, "Borrowing Trouble," *The Journal of American Folklore* 11, no. 40 (1898): 55, doi:10.2307/533610.

17. Tony Tost, "Swans of Local Waters," in *Invisible Bride* (Baton Rouge: Louisiana State University Press, 2004), 33.

18. Amy Lawless, "Elephants in Mourning," in *My Dead* (Portland, Denver, and Omaha: Octopus Books, 2013).

19. "World: South Asia Elephant Dies of Grief," BBC News, last modified May 6, 1999, news.bbc.co.uk/2/hi/south_asia/337356.stm.

20. Isabel Gay A. Bradshaw, "Not by Bread Alone: Symbolic Loss, Trauma, and Recovery in Elephant Communities," *Society & Animals* 12, no. 2 (June 2004): 147, doi:10.1163/1568530041446535.

21. Roualeyn Gordon-Cumming, *A Hunter's Life Among Lions, Elephants, and Other Wild Animals of South Africa* (New York: Derby & Jackson, 1857), 15–16, Biodiversity Heritage Library, EBSCO-host (accessed September 27, 2017).

22. Matt Walker, *Fish That Fake Orgasms* (New York: St. Martin's Press, 2007), 39–40.

23. bell hooks, *The Will to Change: Men, Masculinity, and Love* (New York: Atria Books, 2004), 135–36.

24. Anne Carson, *If Not, Winter: Fragments of Sappho* (New York: Vintage Books, 2002), 287.

25. Tom Lutz, *Crying* (New York: Norton, 1999), 157–68.

26. Ibid., 109.

27. James Elkins, *Pictures & Tears* (New York: Routledge, 2001), v.

28. Lutz, *Crying*, 264.

29. Ibid.

30. Ibid., 264–65.

31. Shirley Temple Black, *Child Star* (New York: McGraw Hill, 1988), 49–50.

32. Harriet Baskas, "Virgin Atlantic Airways Offers 'Weep Warnings' on In-flight Movie," NBCNews.com, August 22, 2011, overheadbin.nbcnews.com/_news/2011/08/20/7426102-virgin-atlantic-airways-offers-weep-warnings-on-in-flight-movies.

33. Mary Ruefle, "On Erasure," *Quarter After Eight*, vol. 16, www.quarteraftereight.org/toc.html#on

34. Jack Spicer, from *After Lorca* in *My Vocabulary Did This to Me*, ed. Peter Gizzi and Kevin Killian (Middletown, Conn.: Wesleyan University Press, 2010), 133.

35. Robert Desnos, "I Have Dreamed of You So Much," in *The Random House Book of Twentieth-Century French Poetry*, ed. and trans. Paul Auster (New York: Random House, 1982), 281.

36. Ibid.

37. June Gruber, "Human Emotion 2.1: Emotion Elicitation 1," *Human Emotion: Yale University Psych 131*, July 15, 2013, iTunes U.

38. Amy Hempel, "In the Cemetery Where Al Jolson Is Buried," in *The Collected Stories of Amy Hempel* (New York: Scribner, 2006), 40.

39. Roger Fouts, *Next of Kin* (London: Penguin, 1997), 280–81.

40. Chris Hadfield, "Can You Cry in Space?," YouTube video, 1:24, posted by "VideoFromSpace," April 8, 2013, www.youtube.com /watch?v=1v5gtOkyCG0.

41. "Rumbles," *Avalanche* 2 (Winter 1971): 2.

42. Anne Carson, "Uncle Falling," in *Float* (New York: Alfred A. Knopf, 2016).

43. Paige M. Lewis, Twitter post, November 18, 2017, twitter.com /Paige_M_Lewis/status/931950473824931841.

44. Temple Black, *Child Star*, 362.

45. J. W. Slaughter, "The Moon in Childhood and Folklore," *The American Journal of Psychology* 13, no. 2 (1902): 297, doi:10.2307/1412741.

46. William Carlos Williams, "The Last Words of My English Grandmother," in *Selected Poems* (New York: New Directions, 1968), 94–96.

47. Carl von Clausewitz, *On War*, trans. Michael Howard and Peter Paret (Princeton, N.J.: Princeton University Press, 2008), 140.

48. Pam Belluck, "After Baby, an Unraveling," *The New York Times*, June 16, 2014, www.nytimes.com/2014/06/17/health/maternal -mental-illness-can-arrive-months-after-baby.html?_r=0.

49. Margery Kempe, *The Book of Margery Kempe*, trans. B. A. Windeatt (London: Penguin Books, 1994), 41–42.

50. Ibid.

51. Ibid., 103.

52. Mathias Svalina, from *Thank You Terror*. Private communication from author.

53. Rachel Zucker, "What Dark Thing," in *Museum of Accidents* (Seattle: Wave Books, 2009), 9.

54. Sylvia Plath, "The Moon and the Yew Tree," in *The Collected Poems*, ed. Ted Hughes (New York: Harper & Row, 1981), 173.

55. Christopher Alexander et al., *A Pattern Language* (New York: Oxford University Press, 1977), xli.

56. Lisa Olstein, "Ready Regret," in *Late Empire* (Port Townsend, WA: Copper Canyon Press, 2017), 83.

57. Harmony Holiday, "Preface to James Baldwin's Unwritten Suicide Note," *Harriet Blog*, August 9, 2018, www.poetryfoundation.org /harriet/2018/08/preface-to-james-baldwins-unwritten-suicide -note.

58. Plath, "The Moon and the Yew Tree," 173.

59. Christina Sharpe, *In the Wake: On Blackness and Being* (Durham, N.C., and London: Duke University Press, 2016), 104.

60. Ashley C. Ford, Twitter post, December 18, 2015, 4:40 p.m., twitter.com/iSmashFizzle/status/681590634084470785.

61. Brittney Cooper, "White Girl Tears," in *Eloquent Rage: A Black Feminist Discovers Her Superpower* (New York: St. Martin's Press, 2018), 175.

62. As of March 2019, the quest for justice for John Crawford III continues. In addition to their ongoing work to hold the police accountable for his death, his family have established the John H. Crawford III Foundation, whose "focus is multifaceted, including educating and supporting families of police brutality. In addition, the foundation continues to work with community leadership and citizens on reforming the criminal justice system, with a specific focus on police accountability, in efforts to stop these egregious acts of violence." To learn more about the foundation, visit thejohncrawfordfoundation.org.

63. Alvin Borgquist, "Crying," *The American Journal of Psychology* 17, no. 2 (1906): 150, doi:10.2307/1412391.

64. Ibid.

65. Ibid., 151.

66. Letter, Alvin Borgquist to W. E. B. Du Bois, April 3, 1905, W. E. B. Du Bois Papers (MS 312), Special Collections and University Archives, University of Massachusetts Amherst Libraries.

67. Lucille Clifton, "reply," in *The Collected Poems of Lucille Clifton 1965–2010*, ed. Kevin Young and Michael S. Glaser (Rochester, N.Y.: BOA Editions, 2012), 337.

68. Lucille Clifton, "reply," page proof with corrections, 1991, Box 19, Folder 1, Lucille Clifton Papers, Stuart A. Rose Manuscript, Archives, and Rare Book Library, Emory University.

69. Charles Darwin, *The Expression of the Emotions in Man and Animals* (New York: AMS Press, 1972), 148.

70. Ibid., 153.

71. Nico J. van Haeringen, "The (Neuro)anatomy of the Lacrimal System and the Biological Aspects of Crying," in *Adult Crying: A Biopsychosocial Approach*, ed. Ad J. J. M. Vingerhoets and Randolph R. Cornelius (London and New York: Routledge, 2001), 19.

72. Michele Christle, "March of the Volunteers" (unpublished manuscript).

73. Charlotte Perkins Gilman, *Women and Economics: A Study of the Economic Relations Between Men and Women as a Factor in Social Evolution* (Boston: Small, Maynard & Company, 1898), 243–44.

74. Kempe, *The Book of Margery Kempe*, 41.

75. Ibid.

76. Ibid.

77. Jan Verwoert, *Bas Jan Ader: In Search of the Miraculous* (London: After All Books, 2006), 1–7.

78. Adriana Ader-Apels, "From the Deep Waters of Sleep." The entire poem reads as follows:

From the deep waters of sleep I wake up to consciousness.
In the distance I hear a train rumbling in the early morning
It is going East and passes a border. Then it will stop.

I feel my heart beating too. It will go on beating for some time.
Then it will stop.
I wonder if the little heart that has beaten with mine, has stopped.
When he passed the border of birth, I laid him at my breast,
rocked him in my arms.

He was very small then.
A white body of a man, rocked in the arms of the waves,
is very small too.

What are we in the infinity of ocean and sky?
A small baby at the breast of eternity.

Have you ever heard of happiness
springing from a deep well of sorrow?
Of love, springing from pain and despondency, agony and death?
Such is mine.

Sunday morning
October 12th 1975

Psalm 30:3 King James version: "O Lord, my God, I cried unto Thee and
Thou hast healed me."

79. Julio Cortázar, "Instructions on How to Cry," in *Cronopios and Famas*, trans. Paul Blackburn (New York: New Directions, 1999), 6.

80. Vingerhoets, *Why Only Humans Weep*, 107.

81. James Tate, "Coda," in *Selected Poems* (Hanover, N.H.: Wesleyan University Press/University Press of New England, 1991), 41.

82. Joan Didion, "On Self Respect," in *Slouching Towards Bethlehem* (New York: Farrar, Straus and Giroux, 1968), 146–47.

83. "How to Stop Yourself from Crying," wikiHow, last modified January 3, 2017, www.wikihow.com/Stop-Yourself-from-Crying.

84. Roland Barthes, "Dark Glasses," in *A Lover's Discourse*, trans. Richard Howard (New York: Hill and Wang, 2010), 43.

85. Michelle Tea, *Black Wave* (New York: Feminist Press at the City University of New York, 2016), 56.

86. "Can the phoenix's tears bring someone back to life?," Yahoo! Answers, accessed February 22, 2016, answers.yahoo.com/question /index?qid=20111217192129AAcJNQY.

87. "Crying . . . ?," Yahoo! Answers, accessed July 23, 2016, answers .yahoo.com/question/index;_ylt=AwrC0F_BGw9a5iUA1mZPm olQ;_ylu=X3oDMTEyNHBhYnJtBGNvbG8DYmYxBHBvcwM xBHZ0aWQDQjI1NTdfMQRzZWMDc3I-?qid=2006072619 0711AAShCMH.

88. Claude Hermann Walter Johns, *Babylonian and Assyrian Laws, Contracts and Letters* (New York: Charles Scribner's Sons, 1904), 321.

89. Louise Glück, "A Sharply Worded Silence," in *Faithful and Virtuous Night: Poems* (New York: Farrar, Straus and Giroux, 2015), 21.

90. Hart Crane, "Chaplinesque," in *The Poems of Hart Crane*, ed. Marc Simon (New York: Liveright Publishing Corp., 1986), 11.

91. Frank O'Hara, "Mayakovsky," in *The Collected Poems of Frank O'Hara*, ed. Donald Allen (Berkeley and Los Angeles: University of California Press, 1995), 201.

92. Elif Batuman, "Japan's Rent-a-Family Industry," *The New Yorker*, April 30, 2018.

93. Olivia B. Waxman, "This Hotel's 'Crying Rooms' Are Perfect for When You Need a Good Sob," Time.com, last modified May 8, 2015, time.com/3850283/japan-hotel-crying-rooms.

94. Franck André Jamme, "to be," in *New Exercises*, trans. Charles Borkhuis (Seattle/New York: Wave Books, 2008), 31.

95. Carl Phillips, "Gold Leaf," in *Wild Is the Wind* (New York: Farrar, Straus and Giroux, 2018), 13.

96. Lorrie Moore, "People Like That Are the Only People Here," *The New Yorker*, January 27, 1997, 68.

97. Douglas Keister, *Stories in Stone* (Layton, Utah: Gibbs Smith, 2004), 139.

98. Edward Fitzgerald, *A Hand Book for the Albany Rural Cemetery* (Albany: Van Benthuysen Printing House, 1871), 58.

99. Joseph Stromberg, "The Microscopic Structures of Dried Human Tears," Smithsonian.com, last modified November 19, 2013, www.smithsonianmag.com/science-nature/the-microscopic-structures-of-dried-human-tears-180947766.

100. A. Caswell Ellis and G. Stanley Hall, "A Study of Dolls," *The Pedagogical Seminary* 4 (1897): 139. Retrieved from books.google.com/books?id=hW4VAAAAIAAJ&source=gbs_navlinks_s.

101. Ibid., 146. (Line breaks mine.)

102. Angelika Kretschmer, "Mortuary Rites for Inanimate Objects: The Case of Hari Kuyō," *Japanese Journal of Religious Studies* 27, no. 3/4 (2000): 379–404, www.jstor.org.ezproxy.libraries.wright.edu/stable/30233671.

103. User name momoftwo, "Baby Annabell Customer Review," Amazon, last modified November 14, 2005, www.amazon.com/gp/review/R2BJHZQJHN34AQ?ref_=glimp_1rv_cl.

104. Anna Leavitt, "Huge Dissapointment! Customer Review," Amazon, last modified November 12, 2005, www.amazon.com/gp/review/R28GUZD3GHRWDL?ref_=glimp_1rv_cl.

105. N. Guido, "Broke after 4 months Customer Review," Amazon, last modified April 7, 2016, www.amazon.com/gp/customer-reviews/RU09SMSXYCYQP/ref=cm_cr_arp_d_rvw_ttl?ie=UTF8&ASIN=B00JA1HTLS.

106. Chris Meigh-Andrews, *A History of Video Art* (New York and London: Bloomsbury Academic, 2006), 309.

107. K. G. Karakatsanis, "'Brain Death': Should It Be Reconsidered?," *Spinal Cord* 46, no. 6 (2008): 399, Academic Search Complete, EBSCOhost (accessed December 1, 2017).

108. Charlotte Perkins Gilman and Denise D. Knight, *The Diaries of Charlotte Perkins Gilman, Vol. 1: 1879–87* (University Press of Virginia, 1994), 344.

109. Sylvia Plath, *The Bell Jar* (New York: Harper & Row, 1971), 82–83.

110. Leo Lionni, *Little Blue and Little Yellow* (New York: Dragonfly Books–Random House Children's Books, 1959, reprint 2017).

111. Plath, "The Moon and the Yew Tree," 173.

112. Brian Boyd, *On the Origin of Stories: Evolution, Cognition, and Fiction* (Cambridge and London: Belknap Press, 2009), 115.

113. Fritz Heider and Marianne Simmel, "An Experimental Study of Apparent Behavior," *The American Journal of Psychology* 57, no. 2 (1944): 243–59, doi:10.2307/1416950.

114. William Carlos Williams, "Asphodel, That Greeny Flower," in *Asphodel, That Greeny Flower & Other Love Poems* (New York: New Directions, 1994), 9.

115. Peter Richards, "The Moon Is a Moon," in *Oubliette* (Amherst, Mass.: Verse Press, 2001), 66.

116. George Lakoff and Mark Johnson, *Metaphors We Live By* (Chicago and London: University of Chicago Press, 1980), 16.

117. Dr. Patricia Fara, Professor Melissa Hines, and Dr. Cailin O'Connor, "Women in Science: Past, Present, and Future Challenges," Public Panel Discussion, Forum for European Philosophy at London School of Economics and Political Science, September 27, 2016, www.lse.ac.uk/website-archive/newsAndMedia /videoAndAudio/channels/publicLecturesAndEvents/player .aspx?id=3588.

118. William H. Frey with Muriel Langseth, *Crying: The Mystery of Tears* (Minneapolis, Minn.: Winston Press, 1985), 12.

119. Ibid., 39.

120. Ibid., 49.

121. hooks, *The Will to Change*, 135–36.

122. Thomas Dixon, *Weeping Britannia: Portrait of a Nation in Tears* (Oxford: Oxford University Press, 2015), 96, 111.

123. "T" is short for "testosterone."

124. Renato Rosaldo, "Introduction: Grief and a Headhunter's Rage," in *Culture and Truth: The Remaking of Social Analysis* (Boston: Beacon Press; London: Taylor & Francis, 1993 [1989]), 171.

125. Ibid.

126. Ibid., 167.

127. Michelle Rosaldo, *Knowledge and Passion: Ilongot Notions of Self and Social Life* (Cambridge: Cambridge University Press, 1980), 32–34.

128. PEN America, "Opening Night of PEN World Voices: Judith Butler," video, 11:21, April 30, 2014, youtu.be/rNmZSROmzeo.

129. "Supercool," *Radiolab* podcast, December 5, 2017, www.wnyc studios.org/story/super-cool-2017.

130. Ami Dokli recorded by Sulley Lansah, "The Women Paid to Cry at the Funerals of Strangers," BBC Africa *One Minute Stories*, 1:00, July 1, 2018, www.bbc.com/news/av/world-africa-44656749/the -women-paid-to-cry-at-the-funerals-of-strangers.

131. Elisabeth Goodridge, "Front-Runner Ed Muskie's Tears (or Melted Snow?) Hurt His Presidential Bid," *U.S. News & World Report*, last modified January 17, 2008, www.usnews.com/news /articles/2008/01/17/72-front-runners-tears-hurt.

132. Paul Rozin et al., "Glad to Be Sad, and Other Examples of Benign Masochism," *Judgment & Decision Making* 8, no. 4 (July 2013): 439–47, Academic Search Complete, EBSCOhost (accessed December 10, 2017).

133. PEN America, "Opening Night of PEN World Voices: Judith Butler."

134. Ibid.

135. Henri Bergson, *Laughter: An Essay on the Meaning of the Comic*, trans. Cloudesely Brereton and Fred Rothwell (Rockville, Md.: Arc Manor, 2008), 12.

136. Rozin et al., "Glad to Be Sad, and Other Examples of Benign Masochism," 446.

137. Laura Varnam, "The Crucifix, the Pietà, and the Female Mystic: Devotional Objects and Performative Identity in *The Book of Margery Kempe*," *The Journal of Medieval Religious Cultures* 41, no. 2 (2015): 208–37, muse.jhu.edu (accessed December 19, 2017).

138. Kempe, *The Book of Margery Kempe*, 187.

139. Zbigniew Herbert, "The Envoy of Mr. Cogito," in *Mr. Cogito*,

trans. John Carpenter and Bogdana Carpenter (Hopewell, N.J.: Ecco Press, 1993), 61.

140. Bergson, *Laughter*, 84.

141. Charlotte Perkins Gilman, *The Living of Charlotte Perkins Gilman: An Autobiography* (Madison: University of Wisconsin Press, 1990 [1935]), 96.

142. Nancy Cervetti, *S. Weir Mitchell, 1829–1914: Philadelphia's Literary Physician* (University Park: Pennsylvania State University Press, 2012), 148–49.

143. Gilman and Knight, *The Diaries of Charlotte Perkins Gilman*, Vol. 1, 385.

144. Silas Weir Mitchell, *Fat and Blood: An Essay on the Treatment of Certain Forms of Neurasthenia and Hysteria* (Philadelphia: J. B. Lippincott Co., 1888), 49.

145. Zachary Schomburg, "Right Man for the Job" (unpublished manuscript).

146. "The goat ate the goat food from his hand," submitted by William, *Reasons My Son Is Crying*, July 26, 2013, www.reasonsmysoniscrying.com/post/56543323715/the-goat-ate-the-goat-food-from-his-hand.

147. Roland Barthes, "November 5," in *Mourning Diary*, trans. Richard Howard (New York: Hill and Wang, 2010), 37.

148. Renee Gladman, "I began the day looking up at the whiteboard," in *Calamities* (Seattle/New York: Wave Books, 2016), 35–36.

149. Silas Weir Mitchell diary, 1898, Box 13, Folder 18, Silas Weir Mitchell Papers, Philadelphia College of Physicians Historical Library.

150. Ibid.

151. In the years since I first spoke with Sharon, St. Stephen's has found new life. A recent email shares the news that "St. Stephens has been open since March 2017 as a mission rather than a parish and ... we have midday services on Mondays, Tuesdays, Wednesdays and Thursdays; music performances; and a community outreach program with a social work student from Temple University." The pool, Sharon tells me, is gone.

152. Frank O'Hara, "Steps," in *The Collected Poems of Frank O'Hara*, ed. Donald Allen (Berkeley, Los Angeles, and London: University of California Press, 1995), 370.

153. Letter, S. Weir Mitchell to John K. Mitchell, January 11, 1899, Box 5, Folder 7, Silas Weir Mitchell Papers, Philadelphia College of Physicians Library.

154. Letter, Alvin Borgquist to G. Stanley Hall, August 28, 1904, Box Box B1-6-2, Graduate Correspondence, Dr. G. Stanley Hall Papers, Archives and Special Collections, Clark University.

155. Letter, George M. Stratton to Edmund Sanford, July 2, 1904, Box B1-6-2, Graduate Correspondence, Dr. G. Stanley Hall Papers, Archives and Special Collections, Clark University.

156. Domino Renee Perez, *There Was a Woman: La Llorona from Folklore to Popular Culture* (Austin: University of Texas Press, 2008).

157. Alexander Chee, "On Becoming an American Writer," in *How to Write an Autobiographical Novel* (Boston and New York: Mariner Books, 2018).

158. Robert Frost, "Mending Wall," in *The Poetry of Robert Frost: The Collected Poems, Complete and Unabridged*, ed. Edward Connery Lathem (New York: Henry Holt, 1979), 33.

159. "Inês de Castro and Pedro I of Portugal," *Stuff You Missed in History* podcast, January 25, 2017, www.missedinhistory.com /podcasts/ines-de-castro.htm.

160. Ibid.

161. Yusef Komunyakaa, "Facing It," in *Neon Vernacular: New and Selected Poems* (Middletown, Conn.: Wesleyan University Press, 1993), 159.

162. Lee Ann Roripaugh, "Poem as Mirror Box: Mirror Neurons, Emotions, Phantom Limbs, and Poems of Loss and Elegy," *jubilat* 21 (2012): 78.

163. Anonymous, "The Case of George Dedlow," *Atlantic Monthly*, July 1866, 1–11; reprinted in S. Weir Mitchell, *The Autobiography of a Quack and the Case of George Dedlow* (New York: Century Co.,

1900) and *The Auto-biography of a Quack and Other Short Stories* (New York: Century Co., 1915).

164. Jillian Weise, "The Dawn of the 'Tryborg,'" *The New York Times*, November 30, 2016, www.nytimes.com/2016/11/30/opinion/the -dawn-of-the-tryborg.html?_r=0.

165. Cervetti, *S. Weir Mitchell, 1829–1914*, 52–58.

166. Aaron Blake, "Donald Trump's Amazing Answer to 'Do You Cry?,'" *The Washington Post*, January 19, 2016, www.washington post.com/news/the-fix/wp/2016/01/19/donald-trumps-amazing -answer-on-do-you-cry.

167. E. Poulakou-Rebelakou, C. Tsiamis, G. Panteleakos, and D. Ploumpidis, "Lycanthropy in Byzantine Times (AD 330–1453)," *History of Psychiatry* 20, no. 4 (2009): 468–79, doi:10.1177 /0957154X08338337 (accessed October 6, 2017).

168. William Cassidy, "tempers & knives," email, 2005.

169. William Cassidy, "RE:," email, 2005.

170. Henk Van Woerden, *The Assassin: A Story of Race and Rage in the Land of Apartheid*, trans. Dan Jacobson (New York: Picador USA, 2000), 5.

171. H. F. Verwoerd, "A Method for the Experimental Production of Emotions," *The American Journal of Psychology* 37, no. 3 (1926): 357–71, doi:10.2307/1413622.

172. Details: Banstead Hospital, Banstead, Hospital Records Data-base: A Joint Project of the Wellcome Library and the National Ar-chives, www.nationalarchives.gov.uk/hospitalrecords/details.asp ?id=43#jump2record.

173. Plath, *The Bell Jar*, 167–68.

174. Verwoerd, "A Method for the Experimental Production of Emotions."

175. Rainer Maria Rilke, quoted in Gaston Bachelard, *The Poetics of Space*, 57.

176. "Automata," *In Our Time* podcast, September 20, 2018, www.bbc .co.uk/programmes/b0bk1c4d.

177. Megan Cook, private Facebook comment, September 24, 2018.

178. "The Green Line (room 11)," *Room Guide for Francis Alÿs, A Story of Deception*, Tate Modern, June 15–September 5, 2010, www.tate.org.uk/whats-on/tate-modern/exhibition/francis-alys /francis-alys-story-deception-room-guide/francis-alys-4.

179. Emily Dickinson, "I like a look of Agony," in *The Poems of Emily Dickinson*, ed. R. W. Franklin (Cambridge and London: Belknap Press, 1999), 152.

180. Vingerhoets, *Why Only Humans Weep*, 14–15.

181. "St. Thomas News," *Racing Junior*, September 11, 2007, www .racingjunior.com/stthomas.htm.

182. Sonya Vatomsky, "Debunking the Myth of 19th-Century 'Tear Catchers,'" *Atlas Obscura*, May 2, 2017, www.atlasobscura.com /articles/tearcatchers-victorian-myth-bottle.

183. Dara Wier, "The Dream," in *In the Still of the Night* (Seattle: Wave Books, 2017), 21.

184. Rob Verger, "Student Scientists Determine That It's Impossible to Literally Cry a River," *The Daily Telegraph*, May 4, 2016, www .dailytelegraph.com.au/technology/science/student-scientists -determine-that-its-impossible-to-literally-cry-a-river/news-story /f02088b2fb6257cd8c877612efc736e5.

185. George Wald, "Eye and Camera," *Scientific American* 183:2.

186. Marissa Fessenden, "How Forensic Scientists Once Tried to 'See' a Dead Person's Last Sight," Smithsonian.com, May 23, 2016, www.smithsonianmag.com/smart-news/how-forensic-scientists -once-tried-see-dead-persons-last-sight-180959157.

187. John Keats, "This living hand, now warm and capable," in *Complete Poems and Selected Letters of John Keats* (New York: Modern Library, 2001), 365.

188. Migiwa Orimo, private Facebook comment, December 4, 2017.

189. Andrea Donna and Natasha Kessler-Rains, private Facebook comments, December 5, 2017.

190. Lev Oshanin, lyrics for "May There Always Be Sunshine," trans. Tom Botting.

191. Thomas Murry and Clark A. Rosen, "Phonotrauma Associated

with Crying," *Journal of Voice* 14, no. 4 (2000): 575–80, doi:10.1016 /S0892-1997(00)80013-2 (accessed November 27, 2018).

192. Carson, "Uncle Falling."

193. Lewis Carroll, *Alice in Wonderland* (London: Octopus Books Limited, 1981), 26.

194. Gertrude Stein, "Sacred Emily," in *Geography & Plays* (Boston: Four Seas Press, 1922), 187.

195. Alexander Vvedensky, trans. Valerii Sazhin, quoted in editor's introduction to *Oberiu: An Anthology of Russian Absurdism*, ed. Eugene Ostashevsky (Evanston, Ill.: Northwestern University Press, 2006), xxii.

196. Danez Smith, "23 Positions in a One-Night Stand," *Adroit Journal* 19 (undated), www.theadroitjournal.org/issue-nineteen-danez -smith-the-adroit-journal.

197. Aram Saroyan, "lighght," in *Complete Minimal Poems* (New York: Ugly Duckling Presse, 2007), 31.

198. Her name, I later learned, was Jessica Smith.

NOTES

Permissions

The image of Mary Ann Vecchio crying out over Jeffrey
Miller at Kent State is included by permission of the photographer, John Filo.

The image of Yi-Fei Chen with tear gun appears by permission of Chen and the photographer, Ronald Smits. © Ronald
Smits Photography / www.RonaldSmits.nl

Excerpt from "Right Man for the Job" appears by permission
of Zachary Schomburg.

Excerpt from "January 1, 1997 (New Year's Day)" from *Letters to Wendy's*. Copyright 2000 by Joe Wenderoth. Used
with permission from the author and Wave Books.

"A woman is cry-hustling a man & it is very fun" from *Poemland*. Copyright 2009 by Chelsey Minnis. Used with permission of the author and Wave Books.

Excerpt from "Elephants in Mourning" from *My Dead*, Octopus Books (2013), www.octopusbooks.net, used with permission of Amy Lawless.

Excerpt from "Swans of Local Waters" from *Invisible Bride*. Copyright 2002 by Tony Tost. Used with permission from the author and Louisiana State University Press.

In the United States and Canada: "142 [friends]" from *If Not, Winter: Fragments of Sappho* by Sappho, translated by Anne Carson, copyright © 2002 by Anne Carson. Used by permission of Alfred A. Knopf, an imprint of the Knopf Doubleday Publishing Group, a division of Penguin Random House LLC. All rights reserved.

Throughout the world excluding the United States, Philippines, and Canada: "142 [friends]" from *If Not, Winter: Fragments of Sappho* by Sappho, translated by Anne Carson, copyright © 2002 by Anne Carson. Used by permission of Little, Brown Book Group.

In Germany: "142 [friends]" from *If Not, Winter: Fragments of Sappho* by Sappho, translated by Anne Carson, copyright

"You should know a 12 year-old boy's murder" tweet appears by permission of Ashley C. Ford.

Lucille Clifton, "reply," from *The Collected Poems of Lucille Clifton*. Copyright © 1991 by Lucille Clifton. Reprinted with permission of The Permissions Company, Inc., on behalf of BOA Editions, Ltd., www.boaeditions.org.

Excerpt from Adriana Ader-Apels, "From the Deep Waters of Sleep," © Erik Ader, included by his permission.

Excerpt from "Coda" by James Tate included by permission of Dara Wier.

"Chaplinesque," from *The Complete Poems of Hart Crane* by Hart Crane, edited by Marc Simon. Copyright 1933, 1958, 1966 by Liveright Publishing Corporation. Copyright © 1986 by Marc Simon. Used by permission of Liveright Publishing Corporation.

"T O B E" is from *New Exercises*. Copyright 2008 by Franck André Jamme and Charles Borkhuis. Used with permission of the author and Wave Books.

Excerpt from "Gold Leaf" from *Wild Is the Wind* by Carl Phillips. Copyright © 2018 by Carl Phillips. Reprinted by permission of Farrar, Straus and Giroux.

Image of Sara Weed's memorial sculpture © Paula Lemire.

Lyrics to "May There Always Be Sunshine" by Lev Oshanin (translated by Tom Botting) appear by permission of Lev Oshanin's heirs.

"lighght" © 1966 by Aram Saroyan. Used by permission of the author.

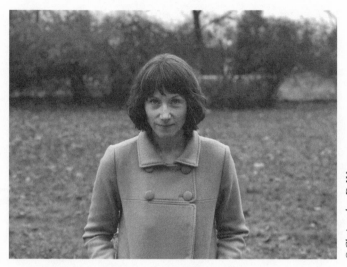

HEATHER CHRISTLE is the author of the poetry collections *The Difficult Farm*; *The Trees The Trees*, which won the Believer Poetry Award; *What Is Amazing*; and *Heliopause*. Her poems have appeared in *The New Yorker, London Review of Books, Poetry*, and many other journals. She teaches creative writing at Emory University in Atlanta.